S0-AHS-553

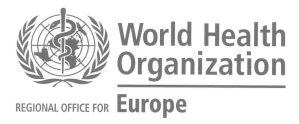

# World Health Organization

REGIONAL OFFICE FOR **Europe**

# Palliative care for older people: better practices

WITHDRAWN

Edited by
**Sue Hall, Hristina Petkova, Agis D. Tsouros,
Massimo Costantini and Irene J. Higginson**

**University of London**
WHO Collaborating Centre for
Palliative Care and Older People

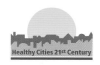

Healthy Cities 21st Century

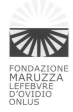

FONDAZIONE
MARUZZA
LEFEBVRE
D'OVIDIO
ONLUS

Cicely Saunders
International
Better care at the end of life

EAPC
ONLUS

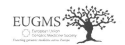

EUGMS
European Union
Geriatric Medicine Society
Fostering geriatric medicine across Europe

Dunhill Medical Trust

# Abstract

Populations around the world are ageing, and more people are living with the effects of serious chronic illness towards the end of life. Meeting their needs presents a public health challenge. This publication aims to provide examples of better palliative care practices for older people to help those involved in planning and supporting care-oriented services most appropriately and effectively. Examples have been identified from literature searches and from an international call for examples through various organizations, including the European Association of Palliative Care and the European Union Geriatric Medicine Society. Some examples consider how to improve aspects within the whole health system; specific smaller examples consider how to improve palliative care education, support in the community, in hospitals or for specific groups of people, such as people in nursing homes and people with dementia and their families. Some examples await rigorous evaluation of effectiveness, and more research is needed in this field, especially the cost–effectiveness and generalizability of these initiatives. This publication takes both an individual person and a health systems approach, focusing on examples from or relevant to the WHO European Region. The publication is intended for policy-makers, decision-makers, planners and multidisciplinary professionals concerned with the care and quality of life of older people.

## Keywords

**Palliative care**
**Aged**
**Health services for the aged**
**Quality of health care**
**Hospice care**
**Terminal care**
**Europe**

**ISBN 978 92 890 0224 0**

Address requests about publications of the WHO Regional Office for Europe to:
**Publications**
**WHO Regional Office for Europe**
**Scherfigsvej 8**
**DK-2100 Copenhagen Ø**
**Denmark**
Alternatively, complete an online request form for documentation, health information, or for permission to quote or translate, on the Regional Office web site (http://www.euro.who.int/pubrequest).

## © World Health Organization 2011

All rights reserved. The Regional Office for Europe of the World Health Organization welcomes requests for permission to reproduce or translate its publications, in part or in full.
The designations employed and the presentation of the material in this publication do not imply the expression of any opinion whatsoever on the part of the World Health Organization concerning the legal status of any country, territory, city or area or its authorities, or concerning the delimitation of its frontiers or boundaries. Dotted lines on maps represent approximate border lines for which there may not yet be full agreement.
The mention of specific companies or of certain manufacturers' products does not imply that they are endorsed or recommended by the World Health Organization in preference to others of a similar nature that are not mentioned. Errors and omissions excepted, the names of proprietary products are distinguished by initial capital letters.
All reasonable precautions have been taken by the World Health Organization to verify the information contained in this publication. However, the published material is being distributed without warranty of any kind, either express or implied. The responsibility for the interpretation and use of the material lies with the reader. In no event shall the World Health Organization be liable for damages arising from its use. The views expressed by authors, editors, or expert groups do not necessarily represent the decisions or the stated policy of the World Health Organization.

Front cover: *Lunch walk on November 13, 2006* © by Joan Teno, Professor, Brown University, Providence RI, USA.
Text editing: David Breuer

Graphic design by Pagina 3 International (Rome)

# Contents

# Foreword

Societies in the WHO European Region are ageing. This produces a need not only to improve health by preventing disease and disability but also to improve the quality of life that remains, enabling people to live well and, when the time comes, to die well. All countries in the European Region face this issue, and the need for palliative care reflects very well the WHO values and principles for dignified, sensitive and patient-centred care for people and their families and caregivers.

This publication builds on two previous publications in the WHO Solid Facts series, Palliative care – the solid facts and Better palliative care for older people, which set out the growing needs of older people, showed some of the problems faced in the European Region and introduced the concept of palliative care. These two booklets have been widely read and used, have been translated into many European languages and have helped palliative care to develop in many countries. However, they lacked specific detailed examples of how practice may be changed. This third publication addresses that gap and is concerned with providing information on the explicit solutions that governments, policy-makers, practitioners and voluntary and statutory organizations can put into practice.

This publication represents the fruits of tremendous efforts over three years. The editors have gathered, from the literature and an international call, examples of promising and best practices in palliative care for older people, particularly focusing on the European Region. They have appraised the examples with an international panel of experts and have ensured that the work is peer reviewed and assessed by experts from many disciplines and countries.

The examples include ways to improve palliative care in various settings such as in hospitals, in nursing homes and at home. There are examples to help support people, such as by improving symptoms, introducing palliative care services – often linked with services for older people – and to support family members and caregivers. There are examples concerned with finding better ways to educate staff in the many places at which older people receive care. Importantly, too, the need for research into the palliative care for older people is raised, since evidence-based practice needs to become integral to the development of services to be taken forward. The examples are taken from all corners of the European Region, and in some instances from elsewhere but show how care may be taken forward in the European Region. The publication focuses on the European Region but may reflect relevant issues in other parts of the world.

The publication targets policy- and decision-makers within government health and social care, the nongovernmental, academic and private sectors and health professionals working with older people. All these groups need to work to integrate palliative care more widely across health services, and policy-makers need to be aware of the proven benefits of palliative care. The publication provides examples and suggestions that will help with this task. It makes recommendations for health policy- and decision-makers, health professionals and those funding research on how services may be developed and improved.

I would like to express my thanks to the Fondazione Maruzza Lefebvre D'Ovidio Onlus, without whose financial support and tremendous enthusiasm this project would not have been realized. I would also like to record our gratitude to Vittorio Ventafridda, who was a key contributor and devoted champion of the publication series and worked towards this third publication before he died in 2008. My deep appreciation goes to all the experts who contributed to preparing the publication, all the services and clinicians who helped by providing examples and to the European Association of Palliative Care and the European Union Geriatric Medicine Society for their technical assistance. Finally, a special word of thanks is due to Irene J. Higginson, Sue Hall and their colleagues in the WHO Collaborating Centre for Palliative Care and Older People at the Cicely Saunders Institute of King's College London and to Agis D. Tsouros of WHO for the effective way they drove and coordinated the whole preparation process and for their excellent editorial work.

I am convinced that this publication will be a source of inspiration, awareness and action.

**Zsuzsanna Jakab**
*WHO Regional Director for Europe*

# Foreword

Improving the care for older people with chronic illness and disability was a goal of Vittorio Ventafridda, founding President of the European Association for Palliative Care, when he called together WHO leaders and palliative care experts to advocate for the publication of a series of WHO monographs on palliative care. His vision was that palliative care would be available to everyone with life-limiting illnesses and fully integrated into health care delivery systems.

Irene J. Higginson was selected as the senior editor for this project and was asked to publish exemplary practices in the care of older people with chronic life-limiting illness throughout Europe. Vittorio Ventafridda also wrote the preface for Better palliative care for older people and subsequently sustained a major stroke that impaired him physically but never deterred his passionate concern for the vulnerability and needs of this ageing population as he lived that experience.

This publication describes programmes that encompass continuity of care for chronically ill older people, focus on their needs and those of their families, provide hospital and home-based care models with sophisticated communication systems and integrate pain relief, symptom control and psychosocial care as well as quality and cost (where available). These efforts vary from country to country and are emerging at the community, national and regional levels.

They demonstrate that the care for older people is now identified as a challenging and growing public health issue. Research efforts to assess the outcomes of older people receiving palliative care and develop an evidence base for the various dimensions of palliative care for older people are underway.

This publication offers a way forward, with numerous examples of care models at varying stages of integration and implementation. These initiatives provide evidence of the innovation and creativity focused on improving the quality of living for this vulnerable population with chronic illness. The recommendations to develop health care policies, educational programmes and clinical and research initiatives frame an approach that can be adapted to country needs, but they clearly emphasize the need for priority to be given to palliative care for older people.

**Kathleen M. Foley**
*Attending Neurologist, Memorial Sloan-Kettering Cancer Center, New York, NY, USA*
*Professor of Neurology and Clinical Pharmacology, Weill Medical College of Cornell University, Ithaca, NY, USA*
*Medical Director, International Palliative Care Initiative, Open Society Institute, New York, NY, USA*

# Acknowledgements

The WHO Regional Office for Europe thanks the numerous organizations and individuals for their efforts in preparing this publication.

**Main partner**
The Maruzza Lefebvre D'Ovidio Foundation provided funding and logistical support for realizing this project and for developing, designing and publishing this book.

**Other key partners**
Other key partners in preparing the publication include: King's College London; Cicely Saunders International; European Association for Palliative Care; and European Union Geriatric Medicine Society. The project was a European Association for Palliative Care task force and worked closely with the European Union Geriatric Medicine Society.

**Editors**
Sue Hall had a central role in the conceptual development of the publication and led the writing. She is Dunhill Medical Trust Senior Lecturer, Department of Palliative Care, Policy and Rehabilitation, King's College London, WHO Collaborating Centre for Palliative Care and Older People, United Kingdom. Sue Hall is funded by Cicely Saunders International through a grant from the Dunhill Medical Trust.

Hristina Petkova led collation of the examples and coordination and contributed to drafting the booklet. She is a Maruzza Foundation Research Associate at the Department of Palliative Care, Policy and Rehabilitation, King's College London, WHO Collaborating Centre for Palliative Care and Older People, United Kingdom.

Agis D. Tsouros had a central role in the conceptual development and strategic approach of the publication, commented on the draft and provided editorial input. He is Head of policy and cross-cutting programmes and Regional Director's special projects at the WHO Regional Office for Europe.

Massimo Costantini had a central role in the conceptual development of the publication, assessed examples and commented on the draft. He is at the Regional Palliative Care Network, National Institute for Cancer Research, Genoa, Italy.

Irene J. Higginson led the project, supervised the booklet, had a central role in conceptual development, contributed to the writing and served as senior editor. She is at the Department of Palliative Care, Policy and Rehabilitation, King's College London, WHO Collaborating Centre for Palliative Care and Older People, United Kingdom. She is also Scientific Director, Cicely Saunders International, London, United Kingdom and a National Institutes for Health Research Senior Investigator.

**Previous Maruzza Foundation Research Associates**
Sreeparna Chattopadhyay and Anna Kolliakou conducted literature searches, assessed examples and contributed to drafting. They were at the Department of Palliative Care, Policy and Rehabilitation, King's College London, WHO Collaborating Centre for Palliative Care and Older People, United Kingdom.

**Maruzza Foundation International Secretary**
Suzanne Bennett provided logistical support and assistance during the production of this publication.

## Contributors

The contributors oversaw the project plan and programme of work, assessed examples and commented on the booklet:

- Elizabeth Davies, King's College London, United Kingdom;
- John Ellershaw, Royal Liverpool University Hospitals, Marie Curie Hospice Liverpool, United Kingdom;
- Mariléne Filbet, Centre Hospitalier Universitaire de Lyon, Hôpital de la Croix Rousse, France;
- Carl Johan Fürst, Karolinska Institute, Stockholm, Sweden;
- Giovanni Gambassi, Centro Medicina Invecchiamento, Università Cattolica del Sacro Cuore, Rome, Italy;
- Stein Kaasa, University Hospital of Trondheim, Norway;
- Lukas Radbruch, European Association for Palliative Care and University of Aachen, Germany;
- Florian Strasser, Palliative Care Centre, Cantonal Hospital, St. Gallen, Switzerland;
- Joan Teno, Brown Medical School, Providence, RI, USA;
- Vittorio Ventafridda, honorary President of the European Association for Palliative Care, Milan, Italy, who initiated the project and identified funding; unfortunately, he died during the course of developing the publication, but the team attempted to follow his vision.

## Reviewers

The following people provided helpful comments in reviewing the publication for WHO:

- Mike Bennett, Division of Health Research, School of Health and Medicine, Lancaster University, United Kingdom;
- Desmond O'Neill, Department of Medical Gerontology, Trinity College Dublin, University of Dublin and Centre for Ageing, Neurosciences and the Humanities and Age Related Health Care, Adelaide and Meath Hospital, Dublin Incorporating the National Children's Hospital, Ireland.

The Regional Office thanks the following organizations who were invited to comment on the manuscript; many disseminated the call for examples and gave useful advice and information:

- European Association for Palliative Care;
- European Cancer Conference;
- European Oncology Nursing Society;
- European School of Surgical Oncology;
- European Union Geriatric Medicine Society;
- Help the Aged;
- Help the Hospices;
- International Society for Geriatric Oncology;
- International Union against Cancer;
- Marie Curie Cancer Care;
- National Council for Palliative Care;
- Scottish Partnership for Palliative Care;
- Sue Ryder Care; and
- Worldwide Palliative Care Alliance.

## Wider consultation group

The draft manuscript was sent to a wider range of experts (Annex 1), many of whom made extremely helpful comments.

## Photographs

We thank the people who provided photographs and other images free of charge for use in this publication.

# 1

# Introduction

Palliative care is an important public health issue due to population ageing, the increasing number of older people in most societies and insufficient attention to their complex needs. Palliative care focuses on improving the symptoms, dignity and quality of life of people approaching the end of their lives and on the care of and support for their families and friends. This topic is often neglected, although it is relevant to everybody. In the past, palliative care was mostly offered to people with cancer in hospice settings. It must now be offered more widely and integrated more broadly across health care services.

Although most deaths occur among people who are older, there is relatively little policy concerning their specific needs towards the end of life. Populations worldwide are ageing, leading to a dramatic increase in the numbers of people living into their seventies, eighties and nineties. Patterns of disease in the last years of life are also changing, with more people dying from chronic debilitating conditions, such as cardiovascular disease, chronic obstructive pulmonary disease, diabetes, cancer and dementia. Since many of these illnesses often occur together among older people, this group frequently experiences multiple health problems and disabilities. In the last year of life, they have symptoms such as pain, anorexia, low mood, mental confusion, constipation, insomnia and problems with bladder and bowel control *(1)*. Palliative care services urgently need to be developed to meet the complex needs of older people. These services need to be available for people with diseases other than cancer and offered based on need rather than diagnosis or prognosis.

This publication is the third of a series published by WHO that aims to raise awareness of the need for better palliative care.

The first publication in the series, *Palliative care – the solid facts (2)*, builds a comprehensive picture of the complex nature of palliative care, describing key trends and principles and discussing their policy implications.

The second publication, *Better palliative care for older people (3)*, focuses on the special needs of older people and the major public health challenge they represent. It provides evidence that the needs

> "All people have a right to receive high-quality care during serious illness and to a dignified death free from overwhelming pain and in line with their spiritual and religious needs."
> *Palliative care – the solid facts (2)*

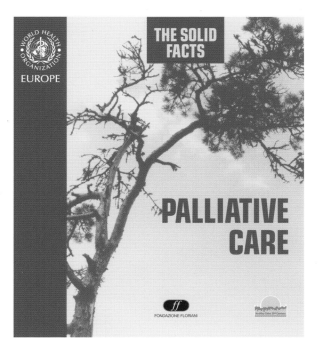

of this vulnerable group are far from being met. Addressing this gap should therefore be a prime public health concern.

This publication builds on the previous two by giving specific examples of promising or better practices in palliative care for older people along with evidence of their effectiveness when this is available. This project is the work of a European Association for Palliative Care (EAPC) Task Force.

> "...older people suffer unnecessarily, owing to widespread underassessment and under-treatment of their problems and lack of access to palliative care."
> *Better palliative care for older people (3)*

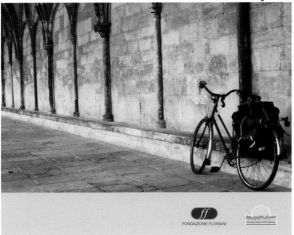

**Better Palliative Care for Older People**

The examples have been identified from literature searches and from an international call for examples through various organizations, including the EAPC and the European Union Geriatric Medicine Society. This publication aims to help those involved in planning, funding or developing services most appropriately and effectively. This guide is developed for countries in the WHO European Region. Where possible, examples from the Region are used. However, some examples from outside the Region are included when these are considered more innovative or more rigorously evaluated than European examples and are relevant to European settings. Palliative care needs to be improved for older people in countries with fewer resources such as those in Africa and Asia. However, the health care systems and the challenges to providing palliative care are very different in these settings, which is why they remain largely outside the remit of this publication. Although some of the examples are not originally intended solely for older people, they have been included because they illustrate care that could also benefit this group.

Many palliative care services provide care for people from different age groups. This publication does not have space to cover many other examples; these are available from the Department of Palliative Care, Policy and Rehabilitation of King's College London (http://www.csi.kcl.ac.uk/palliative).

## Why better palliative care for older people is an urgent public health priority

### Ageing demographics
The proportion of people aged 65 years and older is steadily increasing in the WHO European Region. In 2009, this age group represented almost 15% of the population of most European Union (EU) countries (Fig. 1.1) *(4)*.

By 2050, estimates indicate that more than one quarter of the population of the European Region will be aged 65 years and older. In Spain and Italy, this is likely to rise to more than one third of the population. The greatest percentage increase will be among people aged 85 years and older. Although disability is declining among populations of older people in high-income countries, the increase in absolute numbers means that increasing numbers of older people in almost every society will face the risk of indifferent or poor health care, dependence and multiple illnesses and disabilities. This will also inevitably lead to higher demand for palliative care for this group.

## Changing disease patterns

Palliative care has traditionally been offered to people with cancer, but people aged 85 years and older are more likely to die from cardiovascular disease than cancer (Fig. 1.2). Better meeting the needs of older people in the future requires improving and widening the access to palliative care to include people dying from diseases other than cancer and who have multiple illnesses.

## Complex needs of older people

Older people reaching the end of life frequently have multiple debilitating diseases (such as dementia, osteoporosis and arthritis), and they often do so over longer periods of time. For example, one quarter of the people aged 85 years and older have dementia (6). They may therefore have palliative care needs at any point in the illness trajectory and not just the terminal phase. As such, palliative care should be integrated into chronic disease management. With non-malignant disease, the point in later life at which "really sick becomes dying" can be much more difficult to determine. This is a skill integral

*Fig. 1.1. Percentage of people aged 65 years and older in selected countries in the WHO European Region in 2009 and projections for 2030 and 2050*

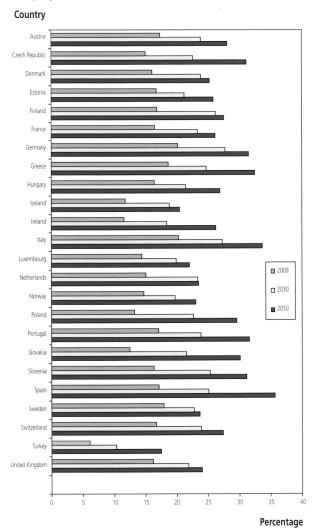

Source: data from *OECD factbook 2009 (4)*.

3

Fig. 1.2. Number of deaths by causes and age group in 27 EU countries, 2006

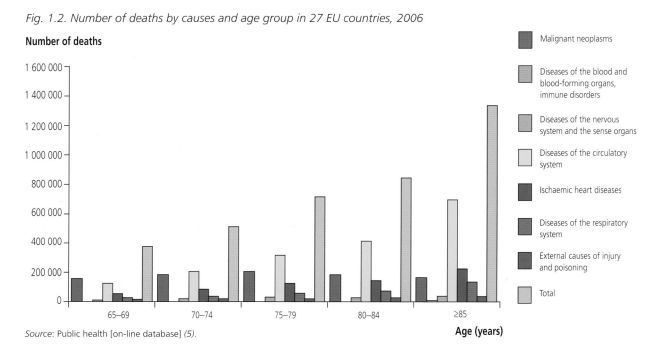

**Number of deaths**

Legend:
- Malignant neoplasms
- Diseases of the blood and blood-forming organs, immune disorders
- Diseases of the nervous system and the sense organs
- Diseases of the circulatory system
- Ischaemic heart diseases
- Diseases of the respiratory system
- External causes of injury and poisoning
- Total

**Age (years)**

*Source*: Public health [on-line database] *(5)*.

to geriatric medicine, other areas of care for older people *(7)* and palliative care. Palliative care is a part of the curriculum for training in geriatric medicine recommended in the EU *(8)*.

**The importance of joint working and interfaces**
The wide range of health needs of older people often requires joint working between many sectors, such as specialists in care for older people and palliative, primary and social care. Both palliative care and care for older people have been relatively neglected in the past and now need to grow and be linked better. Important aspects include:
- the need for palliative and primary care clinicians to receive training in the health of older people and to know about syndromes affecting older

people that are not typically included in palliative care textbooks or terminal diseases, such as urinary incontinence and falls;
- better knowledge about the age-related changes of the pharmacokinetics of opiates for pain management and the polypharmacy (more drugs are prescribed than clinically indicated or there are too many to take) associated with comorbidity *(9)*;
- a holistic approach by health professionals to explore any problems that may reduce people's quality of life, not just those directly related to the life-limiting disease;
- the need for palliative physicians to improve their familiarity with long-term care, such as the administrative and clinical issues associated with older people living and dying in care homes *(7)*;

- training of health care professionals in community settings so that people can be cared for in their place of choice and so that discharge from hospital to home is well managed;
- joint working and new models of integrated care between specialists in palliative care and specialists in care for older people, including training in palliative care for such specialists and training for palliative care within geriatrics.

The EAPC has had a task force working on better practice palliative care for older people with specialists in the health of older people and in palliative care and others, including those working on this publication.

The Geriatric Palliative Care Interest Group founded in 2007 as part of the European Union Geriatric Medicine Society is another example of two disciplines working together. The Group's main goal is to establish a European network of physicians to improve palliative care for older people receiving care.

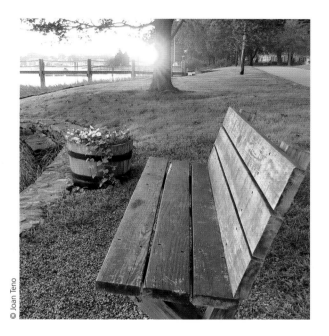

© Joan Teno

## References

1. Addington-Hall J, Altmann D, McCarthy M. Variations by age in symptoms and dependency levels experienced by people in the last year of life, as reported by surviving family, friends and officials. *Age and Ageing*, 1998, 27:129–136.
2. Davies E, Higginson IJ, eds. *Palliative care: the solid facts*. Copenhagen, WHO Regional Office for Europe, 2004 (http://www.euro.who.int/InformationSources/Publications/Catalogue/20050118_2, accessed 1 December 2010).
3. Davies E, Higginson IJ, eds. *Better palliative care for older people*. Copenhagen, WHO Regional Office for Europe, 2004 (http://www.euro.who.int/InformationSources/Publications/Catalogue/20050118_1, accessed 1 December 2010).
4. *OECD factbook 2009*. Paris, Organisation for Economic Co-operation and Development, 2009.
5. Public health [on-line database]. Brussels, Eurostat, 2010 (http://epp.eurostat.ec.europa.eu/portal/page/portal/health/public_health/database, accessed 1 December 2010).
6. Ferri CP et al. Global prevalence of dementia: a Delphi consensus study. *Lancet*, 2005, 366:2112–2117.
7. Finucane TE. How gravely ill becomes dying: a key to end-of-life care. *Journal of the American Medical Association*, 1999, 282:1670–1672.
8. Geriatric Medicine Section, European Union of Medical Specialists. *Training in geriatric medicine in the European Union*. Brussels, European Union of Medical Specialists, 1999.
9. Arnold R, Jaffe E. Why palliative care needs geriatrics. *Journal of Palliative Medicine*, 2007, 10:182–183.

# 2

# Palliative care

## What is palliative care?

WHO *(1)* has defined palliative care as:

"…an approach that improves the quality of life of patients and their families facing the problem associated with life-threatening illness, through the prevention and relief of suffering by means of early identification and impeccable assessment and treatment of pain and other problems, physical, psychosocial and spiritual. Palliative care:

…

- affirms life and regards dying as a normal process;
- intends neither to hasten nor to postpone death; [and]
- uses a team approach to address the needs of patients and their families, including bereavement counselling if indicated.
  …"

Since Cicely Saunders (photograph) founded the modern hospice movement, the numbers of specialist palliative care services, physicians and nurses (those who have accredited palliative care training) have continually increased across Europe *(2)*.

However, the number and scope of services available in countries vary widely, and specialist palliative care often does not reach older people. For example, in the United Kingdom, where palliative care is well developed, the chance of dying in an inpatient hospice declines with age *(3)*.

There is a general move towards offering generalist palliative care, which can be delivered by health and social care professionals, such as staff working in primary care or in care homes for older people, often aided by staff more specialized in palliative care. Whether palliative care is specialist or generalist, services need to be integrated into health care delivery systems to be sustainable.

## Isn't palliative care just good health care?

All the fields of health care that provide holistic care for people with chronic illness are increasingly recognizing the wider needs of older people and their families. Palliative care has focused on controlling pain and other symptoms, defining needs around people receiving care and their families and being flexible about doing what is necessary to help people adapt and cope with their situation. The concept that palliative care is relevant only to the last few weeks of life (when no other treatment is beneficial) is outdated. People needing care and their families experience many problems throughout the course of an illness and need help, especially when problems change or become complex. A more appropriate concept is therefore that palliative care is offered from the time of diagnosis, alongside potentially curative treatment, to disease progression and the end of life. Palliative care is a component of health care that can be needed at any time in life, starting at a low base and rising to eventually become the predominant theme for many people *(4)*.

## The WHO health systems approach

Health systems have three goals: to improve the health status of the population (both the average level of health and the distribution of health); to improve fairness of financing (financial protection and equitable distribution of the burden of funding the system); and to improve responsiveness to the non-medical expectations of the population, including two sets of dimensions, respect for people (patient dignity, confidentiality, autonomy and communication) and client orientation (prompt attention, basic amenities, social support and choice). Palliative care is especially relevant to the latter because it is concerned with the psychosocial aspects of care, dignity and quality of life of individuals and their families. Health systems have four functions: financing (revenue collection, fund pooling and purchasing); resource generation (human resources, technologies and facilities); delivery of personal and population based health services; and stewardship (health policy formulation, regulation and intelligence) (5).

When the health systems approach is applied to palliative care, issues such as the following should be addressed: how health governance should react to the challenges and what needs to be done in terms of legal requirements for integrating palliative care into existing health systems settings; how the funding of health systems can influence options to better integrate palliative care and facilitate the cooperation of health and social services; the human resource implications of integrating palliative care in terms of education and retraining of existing professionals and professions or creating new job profiles; and the expected effects on the organization and the provision of services.

The WHO health systems approach is a holistic way of providing health care services, and it emphasizes the need to be aware of the context in which new services are being introduced: the local health care structure (centralized such as in the United Kingdom versus horizontally delegated such as in Germany); health service provision (general practitioner gatekeeping versus direct access to specialists); funding and human resources; cultural sensitivity; and equity. In accordance with this principle, an example of better practice in palliative care can only be adopted successfully in a system in which it is introduced as part of a continuum of services. This resonates strongly with the Tallinn Charter: Health Systems for Health and Wealth (6), which commits WHO European Member States to improving people's health by strengthening health systems while acknowledging social, cultural and economic diversity across the European Region. To be sustainable, the examples of better palliative care for older people offered here need to be firmly integrated into health care systems. The following characteristics need to be considered when adopting examples in countries.

- The service or intervention needs to be tailored to national demographic, economic, social, cultural and political factors, taking account of the country's health care system.
- The example should be adopted while considering other services and needs.
- The necessary infrastructure may need to be adopted to ensure that examples are transferable from one country to others.
- These examples should be integrated within a health system that provides appropriate, accessible, high-quality, acceptable, culturally sensitive, coherent, consistent and equitable services to everyone in need.

> "How people die remains in the memory of those who live on."

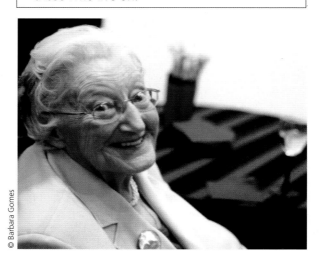

© Barbara Gomes

## References

1. *WHO definition of palliative care*. Geneva, World Health Organization, 2010 (http://www.who.int/cancer/palliative/definition/en, accessed 1 December 2010).
2. European Association for Palliative Care. *EAPC atlas of palliative care in Europe*. Houston, TX, IAHPC Press, 2007.
3. Lock A, Higginson IJ. Patterns and predictors of place of cancer death for the oldest old. *BioMed Central (BMC) Palliative Care*, 2005, 4(6).
4. Lynn J, Adamson DN. *Living well at the end of life: adapting health care to serious chronic illness in old age*. Arlington, VA, Rand Health, 2003.
5. Figueras J et al., eds. *Health systems, health and wealth: assessing the case for investing in health systems*. Copenhagen, WHO Regional Office for Europe, 2008 (http://www.euro.who.int/documentE93699.pdf, accessed 1 December 2010).
6. *The Tallinn Charter: Health Systems for Health and Wealth*. Copenhagen, WHO Regional Office for Europe, 2008 (http://www.euro.who.int/document/E91438.pdf, accessed 1 December 2010).

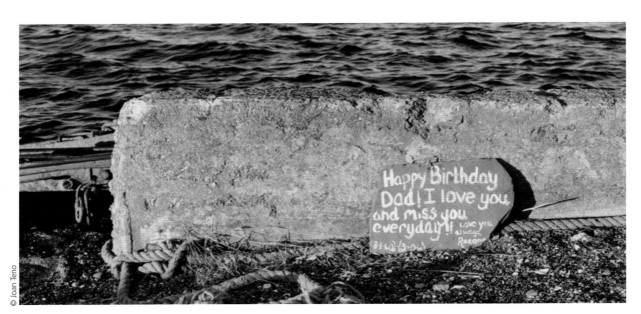

© Joan Teno

# 3

## Place of death

A core value for palliative care has been to enable people to make choices about their end-of-life care and place of death. Most people in the European Region do not die at home (Fig. 3.1), although this is the preferred place of care and of death for the majority *(1)*. Even though some people may change their minds away from home, most still prefer home, even in older age groups.

About half a million people die in England each year. Most deaths (58%) occur in National Health Service hospitals, with about 18% occurring at home, 17% in care homes, 4% in hospices and 3% elsewhere *(2)*.

Analysis of evidence involving 1.5 million people from 13 countries has found 17 main factors related to dying at home among people with cancer *(8)*. The most important are people's low functional status, their preferences, the use and intensity of

*Fig. 3.1. Place of death (home versus not home) in eight European countries*

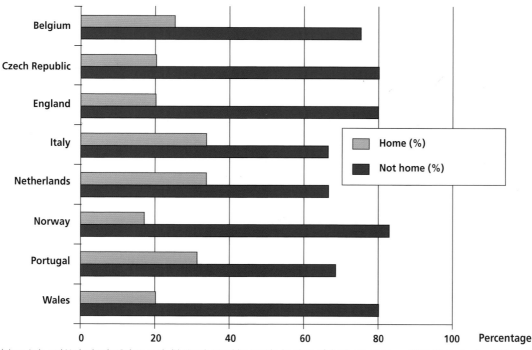

*Sources*: Belgium, Italy and Netherlands: Cohen et al. *(3)*; Czech Republic: *Deaths by place of death, sex and age, 2008 (4)*; England and Wales: *Mortality statistics: deaths registered in 2008. Review of the National Statistician on deaths in England and Wales, 2008 (5)*; Norway: *Deaths of underlying cause of death, by place of death. Per cent. 2008 (6)*; Portugal: *Health statistics 2005 (7)*. The sources of data and classification vary slightly from country to country, limiting direct comparison.

*Fig. 3.2. Factors associated with place of death (home and hospital only)*

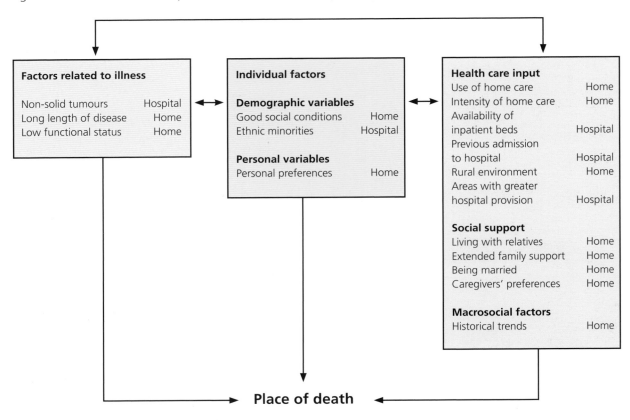

| **Factors related to illness** | |
| Non-solid tumours | Hospital |
| Long length of disease | Home |
| Low functional status | Home |

| **Individual factors** | |
| **Demographic variables** | |
| Good social conditions | Home |
| Ethnic minorities | Hospital |
| **Personal variables** | |
| Personal preferences | Home |

| **Health care input** | |
| Use of home care | Home |
| Intensity of home care | Home |
| Availability of inpatient beds | Hospital |
| Previous admission to hospital | Hospital |
| Rural environment | Home |
| Areas with greater hospital provision | Hospital |
| **Social support** | |
| Living with relatives | Home |
| Extended family support | Home |
| Being married | Home |
| Caregivers' preferences | Home |
| **Macrosocial factors** | |
| Historical trends | Home |

**Place of death**

*Source:* adapted from Gomes & Higginson *(8).*

home care, living with relatives and having extended family support *(8)*. The interplay between these factors can add further complexity. The association between age and place of death varies both within and between countries *(9)*. For example, in London, United Kingdom, older age is associated with a higher probability of dying in a hospital or in a nursing home and a lower chance of dying at home or in an inpatient hospice.

In New York City, United States of America, older people are more likely to die at home or in nursing homes than in a hospital *(9)*.

## References

1. Higginson IJ, Sen-Gupta GJA. Place of care in advanced cancer: a qualitative systematic literature review of patients preferences. *Journal of Palliative Medicine,* 2000, 3:287–300.

2. Department of Health. *End of life care strategy: promoting high quality care for all adults at the end of life.* London, Department of Health, 2008.

3. Cohen J et al. Which patients with cancer die at home? A study of six European countries using death certificate data. *Journal of Clinical Oncology*, 2010, 28 (http://jco.ascopubs.org/cgi/doi/10.1200/JCO.2009.23.2850, accessed 1 December 2010).

4. *Deaths by place of death, sex and age, 2008.* Prague, Czech Statistical Office, 2010 (http://www.czso.cz/csu/2009edicniplan.nsf/engt/4E002A0A64/$File/401909rf06.pdf, accessed 1 December 2010).

5. *Mortality statistics: deaths registered in 2008. Review of the National Statistician on deaths in England and Wales, 2008.* London, Office for National Statistics, 2008 (http://www.statistics.gov.uk/downloads/theme_health/DR2008/DR_08.pdf, accessed 1 December 2010).

6. *Deaths of underlying cause of death, by place of death. Per cent. 2008.* Kongsvinger, Statistics Norway, 2009 (http://www.ssb.no/english/subjects/03/01/10/dodsarsak_en/tab-2010-02-19-19-en.html, accessed 1 December 2010).

7. *Health statistics 2005.* Lisbon, Statistics Portugal, 2006 (http://www.ine.pt/xportal/xmain?xpid=INE&xpgid=ine_publicacoes&PUBLICACOESpub_boui=129520&PUBLICACOEStema=55538&PUBLICACOESmodo=2, accessed 1 December 2010).

8. Gomes B, Higginson IJ. Factors influencing death at home in terminally ill patients with cancer: systematic review. *British Medical Journal,* 2006, 332:515–521.

9. Decker SL, Higginson IJ. A tale of two cities: factors affecting place of cancer death in London and New York. *European Journal of Public Health*, 2006, 17:285–290.

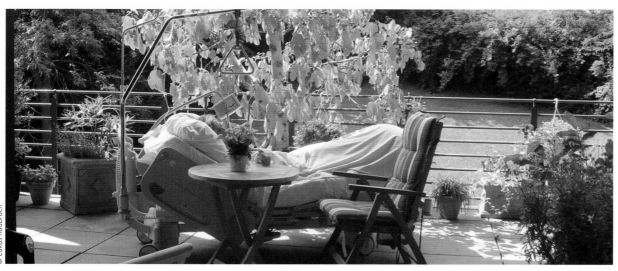

© Lukas Radbruch

# 4

# Whole-system approaches to improving palliative care for older people

To help in developing a whole-system approach or in promoting palliative care, WHO has designated three WHO collaborating centres for palliative care (Box 4.1). Catalonia (Spain) and the United Kingdom are good examples of how palliative care can be effectively integrated into health care systems.

These examples of whole-system approaches include a combination of initiatives (such as education and provision of services) in a planned and integrated way.

### Catalonia

Catalonia has autonomous decision-making in the funding, planning and implementation of health care, which is accessible and free of charge for all Catalonian citizens. Health care services are provided by a mixture of public and not-for-

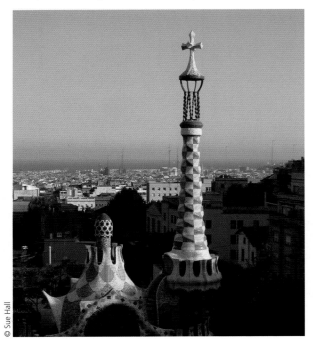

© Sue Hall

profit organizations. The aims of the Catalonian WHO Palliative Care Demonstration Project are to implement specialized palliative care services throughout the region and serve as a model for other countries. The programme is founded on the principle that good palliative care is a right for everyone as part of mainstream health care provision. The focus is on community and home care, and services are available for people with cancer and diseases other than cancer.

As a result of the project, new structures have been developed to provide palliative care services based on the needs of people needing care and their families. Physicians, nurses and allied health professionals work together as palliative care support teams or units in various settings: hospitals, long-term care centres and the community. Services are provided free of charge. The project includes *(5)*:

- revising legislation governing the delivery of opioid analgesics;
- training all health care professionals in basic palliative care;
- developing a model for funding palliative care;
- integrating basic palliative care into conventional health care services;
- implementing specialist palliative care services throughout the health care system;
- developing professional standards; and
- developing a monitoring and evaluation strategy.

With its full integration into the national health plans, changes in relevant legislation governing and providing high quality, culturally sensitive, consistent and equitable services to all those in need, the project meets the requirements of the WHO whole-system approach. Over 10 years, Catalonia's project resulted in a substantial increase in palliative care services, support teams and morphine consumption (indicating increased pain management) *(6)*

(Table 4.1). After 15 years, more than 95% of Catalonia was covered by palliative care services *(7)* and, during 2005, 79% of the people dying from cancer and 25–57% of those dying from other long-term chronic conditions received care from specialist palliative care services. Education and training in palliative care has substantially increased, and a large cooperative research group has been set up. People consulting palliative care teams reported reduced severity of symptoms and were satisfied with the care they received. The resources used have declined substantially *(8)*, including fewer hospital admissions, fewer hospital bed-days, shorter length of stay and less use of emergency rooms. The proportion of deaths at home has increased. The programme in Catalonia has led to an estimated net savings to the Catalan Department of Health of €8 million per year in 2005.

---

**Box 4.1. WHO collaborating centres as a means to help develop plans and policy for palliative care**

There are three WHO collaborating centres for palliative care:
- the WHO Collaborating Centre for Palliative Care in Oxford, United Kingdom *(1)*;
- the WHO Collaborating Centre for Public Health Palliative Care Programmes in Barcelona, Spain *(2)* (see example below); and
- the WHO Collaborating Centre for Palliative Care and Older People, in London, United Kingdom *(3)*.

WHO collaborating centres are institutions such as research institutes, parts of universities, academies and clinical groups that are assessed and designated by the WHO Director-General to carry out activities in support of WHO programmes. Activities of WHO collaborating centres can include: collecting, collating and disseminating information; standardizing terms, methods and procedures; developing and applying appropriate technology; participating in collaborative research developed under WHO's leadership, including planning, conducting, monitoring and evaluating research, as well as promoting the application of the results of research; training; providing support for other countries; and coordinating activities. These three centres are all specialists in palliative care. WHO has a searchable database with further details about how to contact the centres, their activities, annual reports and support provided *(4)*.

---

**Table 4.1. Palliative care services in Catalonia, 1989–2005**

| Services | 1989–1990 (start of project) | 1995 | 2001 | 2005 |
|---|---|---|---|---|
| Palliative care services with beds | 2 | 21 | 50 | 63 |
| Home care support teams | 1 | 44 | 52 | 70 |
| Hospital support teams | 1 | 18 | 20 | 34 |
| Morphine consumption (mg per person per year) | 3.5 | 11.4 | 17 | 21 |

*Source:* Gómez-Batiste et al. *(5,7)*.

### The End of Life Care Strategy in England

The National Health Service (NHS) in the United Kingdom operates under central management from the Department of Health and is funded through general taxation. Health care services are free of user fees at the point of access. Various staff members working in health and social care and the independent sector can provide palliative care across all care settings.

A combination of NHS resources and the voluntary sector funds palliative care. A whole-system and care-pathway approach is a key feature of the End of Life Care Strategy *(9)*. Services are for everyone, regardless of diagnosis and care setting. The themes set out in the strategy are based on the best available research evidence from voluntary hospices *(10)*, the NHS End of Life Care Programme (2004–2007),

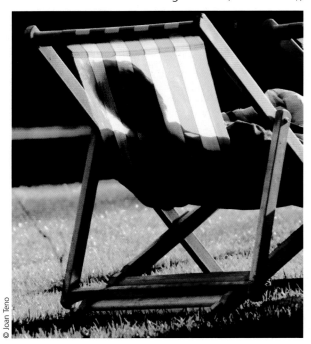

© Joan Teno

the Marie Curie Cancer Care Delivering Choice Programme *(11)* and a large-scale consultation exercise. The End of Life Care Programme included rolling out specific programmes that are built in as examples of better palliative care later in this publication: the Gold Standards Framework for Care Homes; the Liverpool Care Pathway for the Dying Patient; and Preferred Priorities for Care (advance care planning).

The strategy sets out key areas, with related actions and recommendations:

- raising the profile of end-of-life care: working with local communities to increase awareness of end-of-life care;
- strategic commissioning, involving all relevant provider organizations and assessing how any planned changes to services affect their quality;
- identifying people approaching the end of life, including training health care professionals in identifying people reaching the end of life and in communication skills;
- care planning: involving all people reaching the end of life having their needs assessed, their wishes and preferences discussed and an agreed set of actions recorded in a care plan;
- coordination of care, which includes establishing a central coordinating facility as a single point of access through which services can be coordinated as well as locality-wide registers for people approaching the end of life so that they can receive priority care;
- rapid access to care, with health care, personal care and caregivers' support services recommended to be available in the community, 24 hours a day, 7 days a week;
- delivery of high-quality services in all settings, including hospitals, care in the community, hospices, care homes, sheltered and extra-care housing and ambulance services;

- the last days of life and death: the Liverpool Care Pathway, or an equivalent tool, is recommended;
- involving and supporting caregivers, with the family, including children, close friends and family caregivers, recommended to be closely involved in decision-making and to have all the information they require;
- education and training, with end-of-life care recommended to be embedded in training curricula at all levels and for all staff groups;
- measurement and research, which requires measuring the structure, process and outcomes of care; and
- funding, with the government committing £88 million in 2009/2010 and £198 million in 2010/2011 to increase resources to implement the strategy, but many of the improvements envisioned can be achieved by using existing services better.

### The eastern part of the WHO European Region

Palliative care services have developed somewhat in countries in the eastern part of the WHO European Region following the political changes. Some improvements have been achieved with the creation of the International Palliative Care Initiative with the financial support of the Public Health Program of the Open Society Institute *(12)* and following the Council of Europe report on palliative care in 2003 *(13)*.

Nevertheless, services are often unevenly distributed, uncoordinated and poorly integrated across wider health care systems. In the eastern part of the European Region, home care is the most common type of palliative care service, followed by inpatient palliative care, whereas hospital teams, day care and nursing home teams are much less frequent *(13)*. Significant barriers to the development of palliative care in these countries have been reported. These include: (1) financial and material resources; (2) problems relating to the availability of opioids; (3) lack of public awareness and government recognition of palliative care as a specialty; and (4) lack of palliative care education and training programmes *(14)*. A lack of financial and material resources has been reported as the most significant barrier. This has various causes, such as bureaucratic government systems, political instability and pressing social problems.

Mapping of hospice and palliative care services around the world has found that such services are approaching integration in only four of these countries: Hungary, Poland, Romania and Slovenia *(15)*. There are, however, some promising signs of the development of palliative care in the remaining countries (Boxes 4.2–4.5).

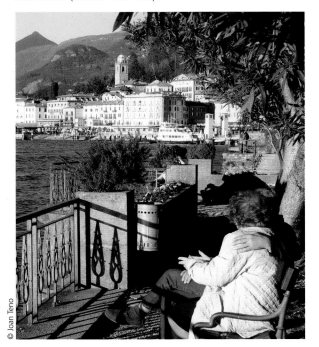

© Joan Teno

## Box 4.2. An interdisciplinary task force on palliative care in Ukraine

Progress has already been made on the development of hospices in Ukraine, and there are plans to develop regional and national programmes, palliative care registers and additional training for doctors and nurses. Access to hospices is not based on prognosis or diagnosis, and they also care for long-stay older people. An interdisciplinary task force, including representatives from both government and nongovernmental organizations, has been created in Ukraine. It aims to raise public awareness of palliative care throughout society, to create patient-centred health care and to develop palliative care legislation. There have been consultations with patients and the general public along with educational events, such as press conferences and films and radio broadcasts about patients' rights and safety. Patient leader groups and information and advisory services have been established. The task force has adopted an integrated approach towards planning and delivering palliative care by reaching out to regions in Ukraine, religious denominations and members of society. Collaboration is in place with other European countries to facilitate the exchange of experience in palliative care. Partners include France, Poland, the Republic of Moldova and Romania. The Ukrainian interdisciplinary task force shows that palliative care can be integrated into a national health care system *(16)*.

*Source*: personal communication, Viktor Serdiuk, All-Ukrainian Council for Patients' Rights and Safety.

## Box 4.3. Humanists Union, a palliative care association in Tbilisi, Georgia

Palliative care is a fairly new but rapidly developing discipline within the health care system in Georgia. Two nongovernmental organizations, the Cancer Prevention Centre and Humanists' Union *(17)*, coordinate palliative care services. Since palliative care emerged in public discussions in 1995, the traditional focus on cancer via the Cancer Prevention Centre has gradually shifted to other incurable diseases (with services currently provided for inpatient care for people with cancer and HIV and for older people in the framework of the Georgian Home Care Coalition); more educational programmes, enhanced awareness about symptom control and pain management and elaboration of the state policy on drug availability. Work is underway to create a national programme for palliative care. The state budget covers 70% of the cost of services.

One main goal of the Humanists Union is to promote the development of a palliative care system and the implementation of internationally approved bioethical standards to underpin the creation and success of a modern palliative care service in Georgia. The Association has partners, collaborators and supporters from a wide range of government and nongovernmental organizations and international institutions, including Georgia's Ministry of Health, Labour and Social Affairs, the Parliament of Georgia, Tbilisi State Medical University, National Society of the Red Cross, the mass media, San Diego Hospice, the Hungarian Palliative Care Association and the Hospice Foundation.

Significant steps have been taken to raise the awareness and standards of palliative care: developing educational material (handbooks on palliative care) for medical students; initiating palliative care as a university discipline; practical training of health care staff members; and creating a mobile team (home-based hospice) providing palliative care to people with incurable diseases at home.

*Sources*: personal communications, Tamari Rukhadze, Humanists' Union and Ioseb Abesadze, Cancer Prevention Centre, Tbilisi, Georgia.

**Box 4.4. Gerontology Institute "13 November", Skopje, the former Yugoslav Republic of Macedonia**

Following the opening of the first hospice in the former Yugoslav Republic of Macedonia in 1998, the integration of palliative services into the health care system has made considerable progress. This includes providing high-quality care to people reaching the end of life in different settings; developing interdisciplinary palliative care teams; ensuring the participation of people at the end of life and their families in decision-making; and ensuring adequate funding through the health insurance fund. The main public health institution for palliative care in Macedonia is the Gerontology Institute "13 November" in Skopje *(18)*. The Institute draws on the Sue Ryder hospice model developed in the United Kingdom. One of its tasks is to evaluate, report and plan for the needs of older people, and it collaborates with several health institutes, clinical centres and a military and psychiatric hospital to improve care of older people with acute and chronic diseases, including those at the end of life. Education in palliative care for health professionals is an integral part of the Institute's activity.

*Source*: personal communication, Mirjana Adzic, National Coordinator for Palliative Care and former director of the Gerontology Institute "13 November".

---

**Box 4.5. Establishing palliative care as a speciality via a state programme in Latvia**

A crucial step in the development of palliative care in Latvia is the establishment of a national programme, which defined a national strategy for the following five to seven years. Palliative care became a part of the Cancer Control Programme in January 2009. The Programme identifies three levels of palliative care: specialized, general and primary. It also specifies the necessary structures for providing palliative care (specialized units, day care centres, mobile teams and home care); educational programmes, human resources and potential financial resources.

Another step forward was made in March 2009, with the government recognizing that palliative care is a separate speciality. These steps helped bridge the gap between specialists and policy-makers and encouraged the introduction of palliative care for diseases other than cancer, targeting in particular end-of-life care and health care for older people.

The state programme stresses the importance of societal awareness and education. It also emphasizes the need for guidelines for family doctors, caregivers, volunteers and other interested people.

*Source*: personal communication, Vilnis Sosars, Palliative Care Unit, Latvian Oncological Centre, Riga, Latvia.

## References

1. Sir Michael Sobell House Hospice [web site]. Oxford, Sir Michael Sobell House Hospice, 2010 (http://www.sobellhospiceoxford.org, accessed 1 December 2010).

2. Institut Català d'Oncologia [web site]. Barcelona, Institut Catalàd'Oncologia, 2010 (http://www.iconcologia.net/index_eng.htm, accessed 1 December 2010).

3. Palliative care, policy and rehabilitation [web site]. London, Department of Palliative Care, Policy and Rehabilitation, King's College London, 2010 (http://www.kcl.ac.uk/palliative, accessed 1 December 2010).

4. The WHO Collaborating Centres Database [online database]. Geneva, World Health Organization, 2010 (http://apps.who.int/whocc/Default.aspx, accessed 1 December 2010).

5. Gómez-Batiste X et al. Catalonia's five-year plan: basic principles. *European Journal of Palliative Care*, 1994, 1:45–49.

6. Gómez-Batiste X et al. Spain: the WHO Demonstration Project of Palliative Care Implementation in Catalonia: results at 10 years (1991–2001). *Journal of Pain and Symptom Management*, 2002, 24:239–244.

7. Gómez-Batiste X et al. Catalonia WHO Palliative Care Demonstration Project at 15 years (2005). *Journal of Pain and Symptom Management*, 2007, 33:584–590.

8. Gómez-Batiste X et al. Resource consumption and costs of palliative care services in Spain: a multicenter prospective study. *Journal of Pain and Symptom Management*, 2006, 31:522–532.

9. *End of Life Care Strategy: promoting high quality care for all adults at the end of life.* London, Department of Health, 2008.

10. Gysels M, Higginsin IJ. *Improving supportive and palliative care for adults with cancer: research evidence.* London, National Institute for Health and Clinical Excellence, 2004.

11. *End of life care: better patient outcomes, genuine patient choice.* London, Marie Curie Delivering Choice Programme, 2009 (http://deliveringchoice.mariecurie.org.uk/NRrdonlyres/8D53D050-A160-475F-9DA6-344ED6ADD9AF/0/Feb09_DCPoverview.pdf, accessed 1 December 2010).

12. *Public Health Program: palliative care.* New York, Open Society Institute, 2010 (http://www.soros.org/initiatives/health/focus/ipci/about, accessed 1 December 2010).

13. *Recommendation Rec (2003) 24 of the Committee of Ministers to Member States on the Organisation of Palliative Care.* Strasbourg, Council of Europe, 2003 (http://www.coe.int/t/dg3/health/Source/Rec (2003) 24_en.pdf, accessed 1 December 2010).

14. Lynch T et al. Barriers to the development of palliative care in the countries of central and eastern Europe and the Commonwealth of Independent States. *Journal of Pain and Symptom Management*, 2009, 37:305–315.

15. Wright M et al. Mapping levels of palliative care development: a global view. *Journal of Pain and Symptom Management*, 2008, 35:469–485.

16. Wolf A. *Report on activities of above-mentioned NGOs in palliative care development in Ukraine (2006–2007).* Kiev, All-Ukrainian Council for Patients Rights and Safety, 2007 (http://www.eapcnet.org/download/forLatestNews/PalliativeCareDevelopmentInUkraine.pdf, accessed 1 December 2010).

17. Palliative Care Association "Humanists' Union" [web site]. Tbilisi, Palliative Care Association "Humanists' Union", 2010 (http://www.palliativecare.org.ge/index_eng.php, accessed 1 December 2010).

18. PHI Gerontology Institute "13 November" – Skopje [web site]. Skopje, PHI Gerontology Institute "13 November", 2010 (http://gerontoloski-institut.com.mk/eng/zapis2580.html?id=43, accessed 1 December 2010).

# 5

# National awareness

"You matter because you are you, and you matter to the end of your life.
We will do all we can not only to help you die peacefully, but also to live until you die."

Cicely Saunders (1)
Founder of the modern hospice movement

Health promotion and public awareness have a key role to play in end-of-life care for older people (2). Health promotion and palliative care are frequently thought to be unrelated concepts (3) but have much in common. Health promotion aims to build public policies that sustain health, create supportive environments, strengthen community action, develop personal skills and reorient health services, especially toward partnerships with the community. This approach enhances collaboration and participatory relationships; recognizes the social character of health, illness and dying; emphasizes education and information-sharing; and requires the understanding that all health policies must be designed for ill and well individuals and that health is everyone's responsibility. These principles underpin the WHO public health strategy to integrate palliative care into existing health care systems and at all levels throughout the society.

Palliative care health promotion activities involve educational programmes in partnerships with communities to foster understanding of their health care needs, the acceptance of loss and dying and encouraging personal and social support at the end of life. Other aspects include recognizing the social character at the core of care and loss; and reorienting health services (such as palliative care, care for older people or bereavement care) towards community partnerships (Box 5.1) (4). Community programmes in palliative care can improve direct service provision by enhancing learning initiatives; this is done in many regions of Australia as part of its strategy for health-promoting palliative care (5). The primary objective of the End of Life Care Strategy in England is to raise national awareness as part of its whole-system approach (see Section 4).

---

**Box 5.1. A state-wide effort to improve end-of-life care in Hawaii**

Kokua Mau (Hawaiian for continuous care) is a state-wide campaign based on a community–state partnership to improve awareness of end-of-life issues and services in Honolulu, Hawaii (6). Education in end-of-life issues was developed, and 17 000 people attended educational events including: 95 policy-makers; 458 individuals from 33 faith-based groups who attended training in care of people who are dying and bereaved; 922 health care and social service providers; 347 individuals in academic training programmes; and more than 15 000 people reached through the public speakers bureau. In addition, an estimated 847 000 individuals were reached through newspaper stories, radio and television shows.

The rates of completing advance directives increased, and the proportion of people supporting physician-assisted suicide decreased. The use of hospices increased.

*Source*: Braun et al. (7).

## References

1. Saunders C. Care of the dying: the problem of euthanasia. *Nursing Times*, 1976, 72:1003–1005.
2. Davies E, Higginson IJ, eds. *Palliative care: the solid facts*. Copenhagen, WHO Regional Office for Europe, 2004 (http://www.euro.who.int/InformationSources/Publications/Catalogue/20050118_2, accessed 1 December 2010).
3. Kellehear A. Health promotion and palliative care. In: Mitchell G, ed. *Palliative care: a patient-centred approach*. Oxford, Radcliffe Publishing, 2008.
4. Kellehear A. Dementia and dying: the need for a systematic policy approach. *Critical Social Policy*, 2009, 29:146–157.
5. Kellehear A, Bateman G, Rumbold B. *Practice guidelines for health promoting palliative care*. Victoria, La Trobe University, 2010 (http://www.latrobe.edu.au/pcu/guide.htm, accessed 1 December 2010).
6. Welcome to the Kokua Mau: Hawaii's hospice and palliative care organization [web site]. Honolulu, Kokua Mau, 2010 (http://www.kokuamau.org, accessed 1 December 2010).
7. Braun KL et al. Kokua Mau: a statewide effort to improve end-of-life care. *Journal of Palliative Medicine*, 2005, 8:313–323.

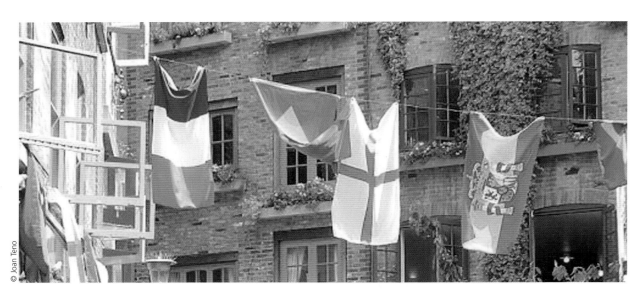

© Joan Teno

# 6
# Educational interventions

A well-performing workforce is a building-block of health systems identified by WHO's framework for action in strengthening health systems, and education is a key component of providing palliative care. An interprofessional, multidisciplinary approach towards learning and communication at all levels of care is needed to meet the complex needs of older people.

Most educational interventions focus on adding palliative care concepts to current curricula for undergraduate and postgraduate medical students. Physicians may lack formal education in palliative care in some countries (such as Ireland). Integrating the principles of palliative care in this way is relatively inexpensive and time efficient. Fewer palliative care educational interventions have targeted nurses, nursing students, nurse educators or other workers (such as care assistants) and volunteers, who are often directly involved in providing care.

The educational opportunities for nurses vary widely between countries, reflecting the position of the nursing profession. Although nurses in many EU countries are able to access some education in palliative care, this may differ between the western and eastern parts of the WHO European Region. Professional health care providers, informal caregivers, people receiving care and the general public would benefit from better understanding palliative care and end-of-life issues. Peer educators could be a cost-effective way of providing this (Box 6.1). One problem appears to be lack of training in managing pain and other symptoms and reluctance to use opioid drugs (when these are available) outside specialist settings. This can be addressed by expanding education and training for staff providing care in all settings, including residential and nursing homes as well as hospitals

and people's own homes (Box 6.2). Another issue concerns the wide variability in roles, competencies and education of professionals in palliative care in countries in the European Region. One way to tackle this is to develop core common curricula for training through initiatives at the European Region level (Box 6.3).

There are synergies between geriatric nursing, palliative care and dementia care skills, which could be further explored for education in the future. Older people with complex needs require combinations of all three and are underserved in terms of all three skill sets.

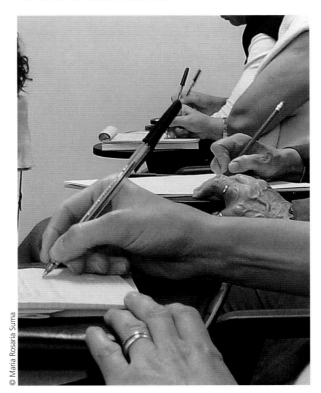

© Maria Rosaria Suma

## Box 6.1. Peer education for advance care planning

This project aimed to raise awareness about treatment and care choices at the end of life among older adults living in the community in Sheffield, United Kingdom. Academic researchers and people recruited from voluntary groups representing older adults acted as community advisers, with some assuming the role of peer educator. A booklet was designed to prepare the peer educators to facilitate learning sessions, covering such issues as bereavement and loss, palliative care and ethical and legal issues. Three days of training was provided. Some of the older people involved appreciated the experience of working collaboratively with other researchers and being peer educators. An extension of the project was completed in September 2009, with 30 people becoming volunteer peer educators. Publications and wider dissemination of the model are underway.

*Source*: Sanders et al. *(1)*.

## Box 6.2. Training the trainers

These courses (MSc, Postgraduate Diploma and Certificate in Palliative Care) have been designed to develop future leaders in palliative care *(2)*. Participants from all over the world develop the skills necessary to appraise research and evidence on palliative care and to improve clinical practice and lead services. The course strongly emphasizes diseases other than cancer and includes sessions on palliative care in nursing homes. A follow-up of career trajectories on completion of the course found increased involvement in a wide range of clinical, research and service development activities, including research, needs assessment, quality assurance and policy development. Participants felt that the course helped develop lateral thinking, challenged misconceptions and enhanced teamwork opportunities, professional networks and confidence and improved their chances of promotion.

Those completing the course then go on to train others in their countries and regions, disseminating skills and knowledge in palliative care more widely. The costs of running the course include a half-time course coordinator, a half-time course administrator and fees for visiting lecturers. Participants have to pay fees to attend, but charities or governments increasingly provide funds for this.

*Source*: Koffman & Higginson *(3)*.

> **Box 6.3. European Association for Palliative Care core curricula recommendations for psychologists**
>
> The Task Force on Education for Psychologists in Palliative Care is an initiative of the EAPC with the goal of developing European guidelines for quality, practice and education of psychologists in palliative care (4). The Task Force aims to gather information about the varying roles, professional identities and education of psychologists in European countries; to define essential competencies for psychologists working in fields of palliative care (such as direct patient consultation, education, management and research) and to develop a common curriculum. This is conducted through needs assessment among psychologists themselves, patients, relatives and staff about the desired support by a psychologist and, finally, a consensus process.
>
> Similar task forces are in place to develop core competencies and curricula for education and training of other professionals, such as:
> - nurses (5);
> - physicians, with a curriculum in palliative care for undergraduate medical education (6) and a postgraduate curriculum in preparation (7); and
> - neurologists (8).
>
> *Sources*: personal communications, Sheila Payne, International Observatory on End of Life Care, Lancaster University, United Kingdom and Saskia Jünger, University Clinic Aachen, Germany.

## References

1. Sanders C et al. Development of a peer education programme for advance end-of-life care planning. *International Journal of Palliative Nursing,* 2006, 12:214–223.
2. Palliative care courses, MSc, diploma and certificate [web site]. London, King's College London, 2010 (http://www.kcl.ac.uk/schools/medicine/depts/palliative/spc, accessed 1 December 2010).
3. Koffman J, Higginson IJ. Assessing the effectiveness and acceptability of inter-professional palliative care education. *Journal of Palliative Care*, 2005, 21:262–269.
4. Education for Psychologists in Palliative Care – an EAPC Task Force [web site]. Milan, European Association for Palliative Care, 2010 (http://www.eapcnet.org/projects/Psychologists.html, accessed 1 December 2010).
5. De Vlieger M et al. *A guide for the development of palliative nurse education in Europe*. Milan, European Association for Palliative Care, 2004 (http://www.eapcnet.org/projects/nursingeducation.html, accessed 1 December 2010).
6. EAPC Task Force on Medical Education. *Curriculum in palliative care for undergraduate medical education: recommendations of the European Association for Palliative Care*. Milan, European Association for Palliative Care, 2007 (http://www.eapcnet.org/projects/TF-EducForPhys.html, accessed 1 December 2010).
7. EAPC Task Force on Medical Education. *For the development of postgraduate curricula leading to certification in palliative medicine: recommendations of the European Association for Palliative Care*. Milan, European Association for Palliative Care, 2009 (http://www.eapcnet.org/projects/TF-EducForPhys.html, accessed 1 December 2010).
8. The development of guidelines and a core curriculum for the palliative care for people with neurological disease – an EAPC task force [web site]. Milan, European Association for Palliative Care, 2009 (http://www.eapcnet.org/projects/Neurology.html, accessed 1 December 2010).

# 7

# Palliative care for older people with dementia

Dementia is a progressive terminal illness for which there is currently no cure. The prognosis may range from 2 to more than 15 years, with the end-stage lasting as long as 2–3 years. One quarter of the people older than 85 years in Europe are estimated to have dementia, with 4.6 million new cases of dementia every year worldwide (one new case every 7 seconds) *(1)*. Although the frequency of dementia in low- and middle-income countries is uncertain due to few studies and varying estimates, most people with dementia live there (60% in 2001, rising to 71% by 2040) *(1)*.

As a result of ageing populations, the number of people with dementia is predicted to double every 20 years, to 81 million by 2040. The rates of

© Catherine Higginson

increase vary between regions, reaching 300% in India, China, southern Asia and the western Pacific between 2001 and 2040.

In the early stages of the illness, most people with dementia are cared for in the community, but more than 95% need 24-hour care as the illness advances *(2)*. People with dementia have cognitive, functional and physical impairment, which gets progressively more severe, often over a prolonged period of time. The most frequent symptoms in the last year of life are cognitive impairment, urinary incontinence, pain, low mood, constipation and loss of appetite *(3)*. The number of symptoms is similar to that of people with cancer, but people with dementia experience them for longer.

The care of older people with dementia is widely inadequate on the continuum from prevention to the end of life. At the end of life, this inadequacy has been summarized as: too much intervention with little benefit (tube feeding and laboratory tests, the use of restraints and intravenous medication) or too little (poor pain control, dehydration and malnutrition, emotional and social neglect, absence of spiritual care and support for family caregivers) *(4)*. There are many reasons why people with dementia do not receive adequate palliative care, including health care professionals not perceiving people with dementia as having a terminal condition and difficulty in prognosis.

The disease trajectory for individuals with dementia is described as a period of "prolonged dwindling", creating difficulty in identifying when people with dementia enter the palliative and end-of-life care phase *(5)*. Communication with people with advanced dementia is difficult, which presents particular challenges in assessing and treating symptoms such as pain and ascertaining their wishes for end-of-life care. Advance care plans need to be initiated at an early stage in the illness to consider personal wishes. Although tools for assessing pain and distress in this group exist, they require detailed and lengthy observation.

Palliative care for people with dementia urgently needs to be improved. Approaches could include interventions for agitation, constipation and pain, which may improve the quality of life, decrease the number of unnecessary investigations and reduce costs (Box 7.1).

As the capacity of people with dementia to make decisions for themselves declines with progression, informal caregivers find themselves having to make difficult choices for those with dementia. Written information can assist caregivers in knowing how best to help the people in their care (Box 7.2). Nursing home staff and health care professionals often lack the specialized knowledge necessary for the palliative support of older people with dementia. One challenge in particular is whether the nursing profession and family doctors recognize these skills as specialist, necessary and beneficial to the care of people with dementia, particularly in nursing homes. Educational initiatives can raise awareness and improve care (Box 7.3). Joint work between geriatric nursing, dementia specific care skills and palliative care will improve all levels of care, as care professionals learn from each other.

---

**Box 7.1. Multidisciplinary guidelines to improve the palliative care of people in the terminal phase of dementia**

The guidelines were developed in the United Kingdom in response to an audit showing that many people dying with dementia suffered from such symptoms as pain, breathlessness and pyrexia. Nurses and physicians working in psychiatry for older people developed the guidelines together with pharmacy and palliative care staff. The guidelines cover managing pain, constipation, dyspnoea, vomiting and agitation, the use of syringe drivers and oral care in this setting. They were implemented in a long-stay unit of a large psychiatric hospital and resulted in a decrease in the prescribing of antibiotics in the last two weeks of life and an increase in the use of analgesia, including opiates.

*Source*: Lloyd-Williams & Payne *(6)*.

---

**Box 7.2. A guide for caregivers of people with dementia**

This guide *(7)* was developed in Sherbrooke, Quebec, Canada in response to the needs of family caregivers for more information on the trajectory of disease, clinical issues, decision-making processes, symptom management at the end of life in dementia, what to expect when the person is dying and grief. It aims to help decision-makers to understand the risks and benefits of care options and to participate actively in decision-making.

The guide is widely used in Quebec, with more than 10 000 copies printed in French and English. It has been well accepted by staff members with many ethnic backgrounds and may improve family satisfaction with care. It has been translated and adapted in Italy, Japan and the Netherlands, and current translation and adaptation work is being conducted for France. This is a relatively low-cost intervention.

*Source*: Arcand et al. *(8)*.

> **Box 7.3. Education to improve palliative care for people in dementia: Robert Bosch Foundation**
>
> This educational initiative for care home staff (caregivers, nurses and head of nursing staff) and general practitioners focuses on improving palliative care in Germany for people with dementia *(9)*. The programme is based on an interdisciplinary curriculum on palliative practice developed by the Robert Bosch Foundation and other experts. It comprises a 40-hour curriculum and is based on action-oriented and practice-oriented learning, including planning care and therapy in palliative support, palliative care for people with dementia, pain management, interprofessional collaboration, symptom control and preferences for end-of-life care. This initiative is currently being rolled out across Germany.
>
> *Source*: personal communication, Bernadette Klapper, Robert Bosch Foundation, Stuttgart, Germany.

## References

1. Ferri CP et al. Global prevalence of dementia: a Delphi consensus study. *Lancet*, 2005, 366:2112–2117.

2. Luchins D, Hanranahan P. What is the appropriate health care for people with end-stage dementia? *Journal of the American Geriatrics Society,* 1993, 41:25–30.

3. McCarthy M, Addington-Hall J, Altman D. The experience of dying with dementia: a retrospective study. *International Journal of Geriatric Psychiatry*, 1997, 12:404–409.

4. Small N. Living well until you die: quality of care and quality of life in palliative and dementia care. *Annals of the New York Academy of Sciences*, 2007, 1114:194–203.

5. Lynn J, Adamson DM. *Living well at the end of life. Adapting health care to serious chronic illness in old age.* Washington, DC, Rand Health, 2003.

6. Lloyd-Williams M, Payne S. Can multidisciplinary guidelines improve the palliation of symptoms in the terminal phase of dementia? *International Journal of Palliative Nursing*, 2002, 8:370–375.

7. Arcand M, Caron C. *Comfort care at the end of life for persons with Alzheimer's disease or other degenerative diseases of the brain.* Sherbrooke, Centre de santé et de services sociaux, Institut universitaire de gériatrie de Sherbrooke, 2005 (http://www.expertise-sante.com/guides-pratiques.htm, accessed 1 December 2010).

8. Arcand M et al. Educating nursing home staff about the progression of dementia and the comfort care option: impact on family satisfaction with end-of-life care. *Journal of the American Medical Directors Association*, 2009, 10:50–55.

9. Palliative care curriculum [web site]. Stuttgart, Robert Bosch Foundation, 2010 (http://www.bosch-stiftung.de/content/language2/html/13157.asp, accessed 1 December 2010).

# 8

# Improving care for older people in hospitals

Although most people wish to die at home, the majority of people in the European Region die in a hospital. Ensuring that older people receive good palliative care in an acute hospital setting is therefore important *(1)*.

Recommendations to improve end-of-life care in hospitals include: educating staff members, identifying and assessing the people who need care, implementing care pathways and ensuring access to specialist palliative care teams *(2)*. Such care has to meet the needs of older people, who often have comorbid illnesses, such as cardiovascular disease, arthritis, dementia or sensory loss and die from diseases other than cancer. Meeting these multiple needs in the hospital setting demands skill and good teamwork between specialists, including geriatricians, oncologists, cardiologists, palliative care clinicians, pharmacists, psychologists, social workers, dieticians, nursing staff, speech therapists and chaplains, at different stages of the illness (Box 8.1). A systematic literature review has shown that hospital palliative care teams are effective in improving symptoms and other problems *(6)*.

It is important to examine how such multidisciplinary palliative care teams develop over time and how they contribute to providing care in the hospital setting (Box 8.2) and as a home care support service (Box 8.3).

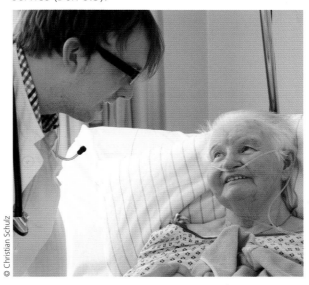
© Christian Schulz

---

**Box 8.1. A multidisciplinary hospital-based palliative care team**

The Palliative Care Team at King's College Hospital NHS Foundation Trust *(3)* is a multiprofessional team comprising consultants in palliative care, specialist registrars, clinical nurse specialists, psychosocial workers and an administrator. The team provides advisory and advocacy services to patients and staff. It complements the hospital services and enables evidence-based, individualized care, symptom control, complex psychosocial care, liaison with other specialist palliative care services (in the hospital and the community) and end-of-life care for people with advanced disease. The team conducts regular audits and is active in research and education. They have a referral rate of about 1100 people per year; 35% of these are for people with a disease other than cancer, such as multiple health problems, pneumonia or sepsis at the end-of-life, dementia, cardiovascular accident and motor neuron disease. This represents one of the largest proportions of non-cancer activity in the United Kingdom. Most referrals are for people older than 65 years.

*Sources*: King's College Hospital NHS Foundation Trust, King's College Hospital Palliative Care Team *(4)* and Kendall et al. *(5)*.

## Box 8.2. A multidisciplinary palliative care team in a geriatric hospital

A multidisciplinary palliative care team has been providing consultation services to the geriatric general hospital at the Geneva University Hospitals in Switzerland. The number of consultations increased from 65 to 100 over five years. The average age of those receiving care exceeds 80 years. The main diagnoses are cancer, cardiovascular and cerebrovascular disease, pulmonary disease and dementia. The team's role includes: pain management, control of other symptoms, psychological support, team support and dealing with ethical and social problems (transfer and returning home). The number of people with diseases other than cancer who receive palliative care has increased since the service started. The team has become involved in care earlier to support home care and to discuss advance care planning.

*Source*: personal communication, Sophie Pautex, Geneva University Hospitals, Switzerland.

## Box 8.3. Home care provided by a hospital-based palliative care service

The palliative home care service at Galliera Hospital in Genoa, Italy relieves symptoms for older people. The service takes a holistic approach to delivering palliative care by means of individualized planning of home care assistance and discussions with the people receiving care and their families. It involves physicians' visits, nurse monitoring and therapy, home health aids, physical therapy and psychological support. If complex clinical situations occur, people can be admitted to hospital or hospice. The service reaches frail older people at risk of disability due to acute or chronic disease and people with end-of-life illnesses (such as cancer or advanced dementia). The service delivers home assistance to about 300 older people per year, of whom one quarter are terminally ill.

*Source*: personal communication, Alberto Cella, Galliera Hospital, Genoa, Italy.

## References

1. Grande G. Palliative care in hospice and hospital: time to put the spotlight on neglected areas of research. *Palliative Medicine*, 2009, 23:187–189.
2. *End of Life Care Strategy: promoting high quality care for all adults at the end of life*. London, Department of Health, 2008.
3. Palliative Care Team [web site]. London, King's College Hospital NHS Foundation Trust, 2010 (http://www.kch.nhs.uk/services/specialist-medicine/palliative care-team, accessed 1 December 2010).
4. *Annual report April 2007 – March 2008*. London, King's College Hospital NHS Foundation Trust, King's College Hospital Palliative Care Team, 2008.
5. Kendall M, Edmonds P, Booth S. *Palliative care in the acute hospital setting*. Oxford, Oxford University Press, 2009.
6. Higginson IJ et al. Do hospital-based palliative care teams improve care for patients or families at the end of life? *Journal of Pain and Symptom Management*, 2002, 23:96–106.

# 9

# Improving palliative care for older people living in nursing and residential care homes

In many countries, care homes (nursing or residential homes, aged or long-term care facilities and continuing care units) play an increasing role in caring for frail older people at the end of life. For example, in England, 17% of the people older than 65 years who die each year do so in a care home *(1)*. The number of older people dying in care homes is almost certain to increase with the ageing population.

Many older people who move to care homes acknowledge these as a last resting place before death. Many develop palliative care needs. Specialist palliative care services may be required for a small number of residents, whereas general palliative care is appropriate for all residents regardless of their diagnosis. When they die, they are likely to have lived with multiple, often-disabling chronic conditions over a long period of time. Common diagnoses include: stroke, cardiac failure, chronic obstructive pulmonary disease, Parkinson's disease and dementia. There are also high levels of impaired cognition, sight and hearing. Many residents experience pain, which is often not well treated and sometimes not treated at all *(2)*. However, the assessment of pain can be complicated by cognitive and sensory impairment. The losses experienced by some residents (such as the loss of their homes and independence) can result in a loss of their sense of dignity *(3)*. Initiatives to improve palliative care in care homes include: the work of clinical nurse specialists, the use of hospice beds in care homes, education and training, the use of link nurses and quality initiatives such as developing guidelines and standards for providing palliative care in care homes *(4)*. Asking bereaved family members for their views on the care residents received can be used to drive improvements in end-of-life care (Box 9.1). Innovative programmes to raise the standards of palliative care by educating care home staff members are being implemented in Germany (Box 9.2) and in Scotland (Box 9.3). The Gold Standards Framework for end-of-life care in care homes is being rolled out in the United Kingdom (Box 9.4). Guidelines are also in place for a palliative approach to care in such institutions in Australia (Box 9.5). A European Association for Palliative Care task force has been developed to identify and map the different ways of developing palliative care in long-term care settings *(5)*.

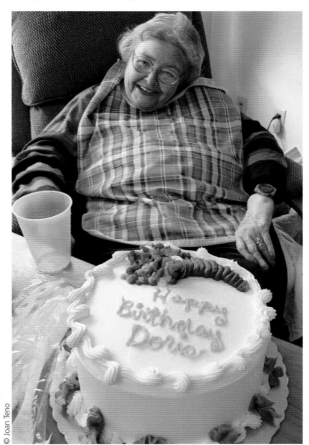

© Joan Teno

### Box 9.1. A quality improvement programme for assessing end-of-life care in care homes

This quality improvement programme was initiated in a United States Veterans Health Administration nursing home in the United States of America. Veterans' homes are primarily for men and are funded by both government and nongovernmental contributions. Representatives of residents who had died in the previous year were asked to complete questionnaires. These included questions on the symptoms the residents experienced in the last three months of life. Plans for improvements were developed based on the representatives' responses.

This resulted in a four-fold increase in spiritual care and a decrease in the prevalence of symptoms such as pain, breathlessness and uncomfortable symptoms of dying (22%, 25% and 30% respectively). The survey took about 16 hours to format, mail and compile and cost US$ 130 for paper and postage.

*Source*: Vandenburg et al. *(6)*.

### Box 9.2. Training in end-of-life care in care homes in Bavaria, Germany

Inneren Mission München is a mid-size welfare organization that has established a training programme Life until the End for health care professionals in care homes *(7)*. The aim is to introduce the principles of palliative care into care homes and to raise the standards of service. This is achieved by educating nurses and cooperating with doctors, churches, hospice groups and palliative care units in hospitals. Staff members undergo training in the principles of palliative care and ethical counselling. As a result of the success of the programme in seven care homes in and around Munich, it is being rolled out across all of Bavaria.

*Source*: personal communication, Frank Kittelberger, Inneren Mission München, Germany.

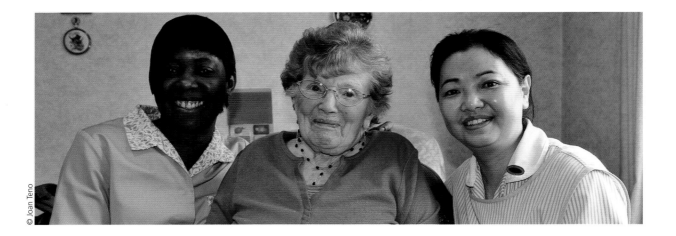

© Joan Teno

### Box 9.3. Training in end-of-life care in Scotland

The project involves training care home staff, mainly caregivers and staff from day care centres for older people, in the principles of palliative care. This includes the physical, mental and spiritual needs of the residents and their families. The project is the result of collaboration between older people's services, social work, residential homes (initially eight care homes and four day care centres) and a care home liaison team. The team facilitates the implementation of the training pack Foundations in Palliative Care developed previously by Macmillan Nurses. The programme consists of four modules (one per week), evaluations by participants and adaptation. Implementation is planned to cover all care home staff in Lanarkshire.

*Source*: personal communication, Ann Hamilton, National Health Service Lanarkshire, Scotland.

### Box 9.4. The Gold Standards Framework for care homes

The Gold Standards Framework for care homes *(8)* is part of the End of Life Care Programme in the United Kingdom. It is a framework of enabling tools, tasks and resources used in care homes for older people, with training and central support from the Gold Standards Framework team and local support from facilitators. The focus is on organizing and improving the quality of care for care home residents in the last year of life in collaboration with primary care and specialist palliative care teams and reducing the number of residents being transferred to hospital in the last week of life. The framework is adapted to meet local needs. To date, the framework has been developed and implemented over five phases. An observational evaluation of the first large-scale roll-out showed a reduction in hospital deaths from 18% to 11%. Examples of potential cost savings in pilot homes, using a sample size of 437 people getting care, include: (1) decreased crisis hospital admissions (12%); and (2) decreased hospital deaths (8%), which potentially equals an estimated saving to the National Health Service of about £40000–80000 per care home per year depending on home size, turnover and tariffs *(9)*.

*Source*: Badger et al. *(10)*.

### Box 9.5. Guidelines for a palliative approach in residential aged care, Australia

In recognition that a palliative approach has much to offer residents in care homes and their families, the Australian Palliative Residential Aged Care project team produced evidence-based guidelines to provide support and guidance for the delivery of a palliative approach in the 3000 residential aged care facilities across Australia *(11)*. The guidelines incorporate the best scientific evidence available regarding all facets of this approach, including the early identification and treatment of physical, cultural, psychological, social and spiritual needs. Guideline topics include: place and provider of care; dignity and quality of life; advance care planning; advanced dementia; pain management; fatigue; nutrition; hydration; cachexia; mouth care; bowel care; complementary therapies; psychological and family support; Aboriginal and Torres Strait Islander issues; and the role of management.

*Source*: Australian Palliative Residential Aged Care (APRAC) Project, Edith Cowan University *(11)*.

## References

1. *End of Life Care Strategy: promoting high quality care for all adults at the end of life.* London, Department of Health, 2008.

2. *Pain in residential aged care facilities: management strategies.* New Sydney, Australian Pain Society, 2005.

3. Hall S, Longhurst SL, Higginson IJH. Living and dying with dignity: a qualitative study of the views of older people in nursing homes. *Age & Ageing*, 2009, 38:411–416.

4. Froggatt KA et al. End-of-life care in long-term care settings for older people. *International Journal of Older People Nursing*, 2006, 1:45–50.

5. EAPC projects or taskforces: palliative care in long-term care settings for older people [web site]. Brussels, European Association for Palliative Care, 2010 (http://www.eapcnet.org/projects/Long-termCare.html, accessed 1 December 2010).

6. Vandenberg EV, Tvrdik A, Keller BK. Use of the quality improvement process in assessing end-of-life care in the nursing home. *Journal of the American Medical Directors Association*, 2006, 7(Suppl. 3):S81–S87.

7. Leben bis zuletzt [web site]. Munich, Inneren Mission München, 2010 (http://www.im-muenchen1.de/pflegeheime/hospizprojekt/s1/index.php?mid=1, accessed 1 December 2010).

8. GSF in care homes [web site]. Walsall, National Gold Standards Framework Centre, 2010 (http://www.goldstandardsframework.nhs.uk/GSFCareHomes, accessed 1 December 2010).

9. Thomas K and GSF Central Team. *Briefing paper on the Gold Standards Framework in care homes (GSFCH) programme.* Walsall, National Gold Standards Framework Centre, 2007.

10. Badger F, Thomas K, Clifford C. Raising standards for elderly people dying in care homes. *European Journal of Palliative Care,* 2007,14:238–241.

11. Australian Palliative Residential Aged Care (APRAC) Project, Edith Cowan University. *Guidelines for a palliative approach in residential aged care: enhanced version.* Canberra, National Palliative Care Programme, Commonwealth of Australia, 2006 (http://www.nhmrc.gov.au/_files_nhmrc/file/publications/synopses/pc29.pdf, accessed 1 December 2010).

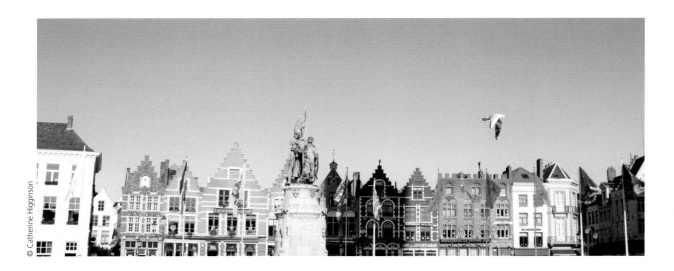

© Catherine Higginson

# 10

# Improving palliative care for older people at home

Most older people in the European Region prefer to be cared for and die at home towards the end of life *(1,2)*. This preference, however, remains still largely unmet. Despite efforts in some countries to improve opportunities for people to die at home, the historical trend toward the hospitalization of death continues, and most older people in Europe die in hospitals or in long-term care facilities (Fig. 3.1). Research shows a steady shift from death in the community to death in institutions, with people older than 85 years accounting for the largest rise in hospital and care-home deaths *(3)*.

In many countries in the eastern and southern parts of the WHO European Region, the lack of state-funded infrastructure for the care of older people may place a greater burden of care on families. Informal caregivers are often not equipped to manage pain and control other symptoms, and people's needs are therefore not likely to be met at home. The reluctance of family doctors to make home visits is an additional challenge.

Promising initiatives have been developed to support individuals dying at home and their families, including specialist palliative care home care teams (Box 10.1) and nurse-led schemes (Box 10.2). To increase high-quality care at home until the end of life, services and policy-makers should develop initiatives that address the areas in the evidence-based model (Fig. 3.2), including providing intensive home support, support for the family and assessing and addressing risk factors *(7)*.

A meta analysis of palliative care and home care teams showed these were of benefit *(8,9)* confirming other reviews *(10–12)*. In addition to palliative care, the many older people who live alone at home also need good health and social care, regardless of their current health needs.

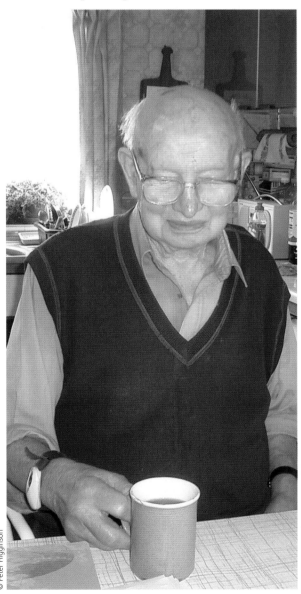

© Peter Higginson

### Box 10.1. A palliative care home intervention

This multidisciplinary approach to the needs of people at the end of life involves a family physician and a community nurse with support in the form of coordination, supervision, advice and visits at home from a specialist palliative medicine unit. It includes an educational scheme for community staff and joint discharge and treatment plans.

A randomized trial of this intervention showed that 25% of those who received it died at home versus 15% in the control group. The service also led to fewer people being admitted to nursing homes. It was suggested that further improvements could be achieved with a more extensively trained home-care team that provides 24-hour service and takes full responsibility for treatment. This approach would address the problem of the limited resources for community services, would help to avoid unnecessary use of high-cost hospital facilities and would eventually increase the proportion of days people are cared for at home. Home palliative care has been systematically reviewed (8–12).

*Source*: Jordhøy et al. (4).

### Box 10.2. The Marie Curie Delivering Choice Programme, United Kingdom

Marie Curie Cancer Care is a charity providing services that aim to enable people with terminal illnesses to be cared for and die at home (5). It promotes care in the community and involves better planning, coordination and uptake of existing local services, working in partnership with local organizations to apply best practices in health and social care. The project currently runs six schemes across different areas in the United Kingdom. The main tools are rapid response teams and discharge community link nurses. The rapid response teams provide both planned and emergency visits to people in their homes during twilight (15:00–22:30) and out-of-hours periods (22:00–07:00), along with psychological support and guidance to people needing care and their caregivers over the telephone.

The discharge community link nurses facilitate rapid discharge of people receiving palliative care with complex needs to their preferred place of care by coordinating home care, supporting and advising these people and their caregivers, communicating the needs of people receiving palliative care to community health care teams and accompanying people home to help them get settled. In the first year (2007), the proportion of home deaths increased from 19% to 23%. The project in Lincolnshire significantly increased the proportion of deaths at home without any additional overall costs.

*Source*: Addicott & Dewar (6).

## References

1. Higginson IJ, Sen-Gupta GJA. Place of care in advanced cancer: a qualitative systematic literature review of patient preferences. *Journal of Palliative Medicine*, 2000, 3:287–300.

2. Davies E, Higginson IJ. *Better palliative care for older people*. Copenhagen, WHO Regional Office for Europe, 2004 (http://www.euro.who.int/InformationSources/Publications/Catalogue/20050118_1, accessed 1 December 2010).

3. Ahmad S, O'Mahony MS. Where older people die: a retrospective population-based study. *Quarterly Journal of Medicine*, 2005, 98:865–870.

4. Jordhøy MS et al. A palliative-care intervention and death at home: a cluster randomised trial. *Lancet*, 2000, 356:888–893.

5. About the Marie Curie Delivering Choice Programme [web site]. London, Marie Curie Delivering Choice Programme, 2010 (http://deliveringchoice.mariecurie.org.uk/about_the_delivering_choice_programme, accessed 1 December 2010).

6. Addicott R, Dewar S. *Improving choice at end of life: a descriptive analysis of the impact and costs of the Marie Curie Delivering Choice Programme in Lincolnshire*. London, King's Fund, 2008.

7. Gomes B, Higginson IJ. Factors influencing death at home in terminally ill patients with cancer: systematic review. *British Medical Journal,* 2006; 332:515–521.

8. Finlay IG et al. Palliative care in hospital, hospice, at home: results from a systematic review. *Annals of Oncology*, 2002, 13:257–264.

9. Higginson IJ et al. Is there evidence that palliative care teams alter end of life experiences of patients and their caregivers? *Journal of Pain and Symptom Management,* 2003, 25:150–168.

10. Hearn J, Higginson IJ. Do specialist palliative care teams improve outcomes for cancer patients? A systematic literature review of the evidence. *Palliative Medicine*, 1998, 12:317–332.

11. Gysels M, Higginson IJ. *Improving supportive and palliative care for adults with cancer: research evidence*. London, National Institute for Health and Clinical Excellence, 2004 (http://guidance.nice.org.uk/index.jsp?action=download&o=28818, accessed 1 December 2010).

12. Smith TJ, Cassel JB. Cost and non-clinical outcomes of palliative care. *Journal of Pain and Symptom Management*, 2009, 38:32–44.

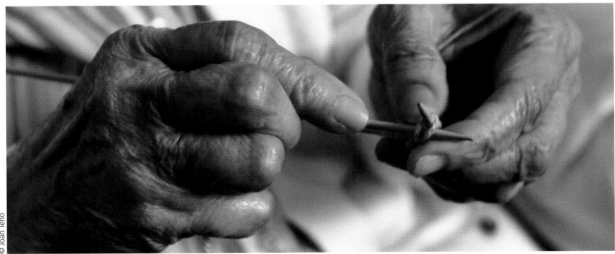

© Joan Teno

# 11

# Family caregivers

The philosophy of palliative care is that the person receiving palliative care and his or her family comprise the unit of care. Supporting the family is therefore a key part of palliative care. Family caregivers can provide help with personal care along with emotional, social and financial support. They often perform tasks that used to be performed by qualified nurses, such as assessing and managing symptoms and giving medication *(1)*.

The availability of informal caregivers is a key factor in determining whether older people are cared for and die at home if they want to *(2)*. In some cultures in the European Region, especially southern countries such as Spain and south-eastern countries such as Bulgaria, caring for older members of the family at home is considered the norm. Older people remain at home, where they are cared for by their family, usually women. However, family sizes are decreasing, and a larger proportion of middle-aged women (who have traditionally performed the role as caregivers) are in full-time employment.

Caregiving can be rewarding when caregivers feel that they have improved the quality of life for a loved one *(3)*. Sometimes, however, the burden can result in physical and emotional exhaustion, conflicting emotions, restrictions on the caregiver's own life and a strain on financial resources. Further, caregivers are often older people with health problems of their own.

Despite the importance of informal caregivers, relatively few interventions have been aimed at specifically supporting them *(4)*. Palliative care services tend to focus primarily on the people reaching the end of life, and the extent to which they help informal caregivers is sometimes not clear. Understanding the factors that influence the informal caregivers' ability to cope with their role is an important step towards informing policy-makers, clinicians and nurses to help reduce the burden associated with caregiving. This includes designing educational programmes or training initiatives specifically for caregivers to enhance their knowledge and confidence and to ease difficulty in caring for older people at home (Box 11.1).

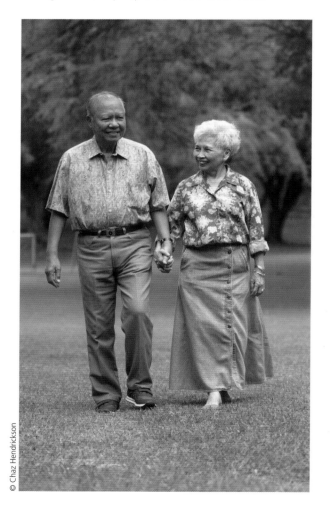

© Chaz Hendrickson

Financial help, such as the paid compassionate leave from work introduced in Canada, may also help to reduce the burden of informal caregiving (5,6). Family caregivers in Canada can receive up to 55% of their average insured earnings over a six-week period to enable them to care for a family member.

Other national programmes for financial compensation of informal caregivers exist in Australia, France, Germany, Israel, Norway, the Netherlands, Sweden, the United Kingdom and the United States of America.

They include:
- direct financial compensation: salary, wages, allowances and vouchers;
- indirect compensation: third-party payment of pension credits or insurance premiums or tax relief; and
- labour policy: paid leave from work, income support or replacement and establishing job security.

---

**Box 11.1. A group programme for family caregivers**

A programme developed by a group in Victoria (Australia) prepares family caregivers to support someone with advanced cancer at home. The three weekly 1.5-hour group sessions involve a mix of presentations, group work and question-and-answer sessions. Caregivers found that this helped to prepare them for the caring role, and most reported positive changes in their lives. The programme makes efficient use of available multidisciplinary specialist palliative staff and can be readily integrated into practice with minimal extra resources. The approximate time commitment for the facilitator for an intervention is one day per week for five weeks. The programme is currently being evaluated in the United Kingdom.

*Source*: Hudson et al. *(7)*.

---

### References

1. Hoffmann RL, Mitchell AM. Caregiver burden: historical development. *Nursing Forum*, 1998, 33(4):5–12.
2. Gomes B, Higginson IJ. Factors influencing death at home in terminally ill patients with cancer: systematic review. *British Medical Journal*, 2006, 332:515–521.
3. Cohen CA, Colantonio A, Vernich L. Positive aspects of caregiving: rounding out the caregiver experience. *International Journal of Geriatric Psychiatry,* 2002, 17:184–188.
4. Harding R, Higginson IJ. What is the best way to help caregivers in cancer and palliative care? A systematic literature review of interventions and their effectiveness. *Palliative Medicine,* 2003, 17:63–74.
5. Williams A et al. Canada's compassionate care benefit: views of family caregivers in chronic illness. *International Journal of Palliative Nursing*, 2006, 12:438–445.
6. Keefe J, Fancey P, White S. *Consultation on financial compensation initiatives for family caregivers of dependent adults – final report.* Halifax, Mount Saint Vincent University, 2005 (http://www.msvu.ca/mdcaging/pdfs/consultation exec_summary english.pdf, accessed 1 December 2010).
7. Hudson P et al. Evaluation of a psycho-educational group programme for family caregivers in home-based palliative care. *Palliative Medicine*, 2008, 22:270–280.

# 12

# Symptom-specific interventions

Physical and psychosocial symptoms are a major burden for people in the final stages of life and can significantly reduce their quality of life. The assessment and management of symptoms is one of the foremost goals of palliative care, and there is major evidence-based literature on how to manage symptoms *(1–3)*. Some symptoms can be highly prevalent across different diseases; others vary. For example, more than half the people with end-stage cancer, HIV disease, heart disease, chronic obstructive pulmonary disease or kidney disease experience pain, breathlessness and fatigue *(4)*. Difficulty in swallowing is a particularly troubling symptom in the palliative care of people who have had strokes or have other disorders of the nervous system. People often have many symptoms simultaneously, and the presence of one symptom can influence the intensity of others. The disease, its treatment or comorbidity may cause symptoms.

The prevalence of cognitive impairment, problems with bladder and bowel control, vision and hearing impairment and dizziness all greatly increase with age *(5)*. The Panel on Persistent Pain in Older Persons of the American Geriatrics Society *(6)* found that 25–50% of older people living in the community have major pain problems, and 45–80% of nursing home residents have substantial pain that is undertreated. Since older people commonly have multiple health problems (including arthritis and other bone joint and back problems), they often have several sources of pain.

The most reliable reports of pain are those that come from the people experiencing the pain. However, older people may be reluctant to report pain because they expect that symptoms are a "natural" part of ageing and do not believe their pain can be alleviated. The high prevalence of sensory and cognitive impairment among frail older people makes communication and therefore the assessment of pain and other symptoms difficult. However, effective ways of assessing pain among people with severe cognitive problems have been developed (Box 12.1). Although older people are generally more susceptible to adverse drug reactions, they can use analgesic and pain-modulating drugs safely and effectively *(6)*. A palliative approach to controlling distressing symptoms at the very end of life can be used successfully with very old people

---

**Box 12.1. A tool for assessing discomfort among people with advanced dementia**

As dementia progresses, nonverbal cues become more important in pain assessment. A protocol for assessing discomfort in dementia was developed as part of a larger pain management project in long-term care facilities in Wisconsin, United States of America. Nurses were trained in assessing pain among cognitively impaired residents, analgesic pharmacology and incorporating the new protocol into the procedures in their facilities. They assessed physical causes for discomfort, looked at the resident's history and took appropriate measures to alleviate the problem or consult with other health care providers. Non-pharmaceutical comfort interventions were used if the source of discomfort was not physical (such as music therapy or therapeutic massage). If these were unsuccessful, non-opioid analgesics were used. Using the protocol reduced behavioural symptoms and increased the use of scheduled analgesics and non-pharmaceutical comfort interventions, indicating improved pain management.

*Source*: Kovach et al. *(10)*.

(Box 12.2). Several drugs can often be discontinued without significant effects on mortality, morbidity and the quality of life (Box 12.3) (7,8). A major barrier to improving palliative care in some countries is the unavailability of opioids. This is a particular problem in some countries in the eastern part of the WHO European Region (9).

The use of multiple medications among older people has increased the rate of drug interactions and hospitalization secondary to drug-related problems. Polypharmacy means that more drugs are prescribed than clinically indicated (8) or all prescribed medications are clinically indicated but there are too many to take. This can potentially cause a higher incidence of adverse drug reactions. The clinical and financial effects of this are enormous and still insufficiently studied.

Increasing age among older people and advanced and terminal disease are associated with changes in pharmacokinetics and pharmacodynamics. Appropriate prescribing in this age group and/or condition can be problematic. This is also an area in which interface, skills exchange and collaboration between specialties may be beneficial in addressing problems and may be necessary.

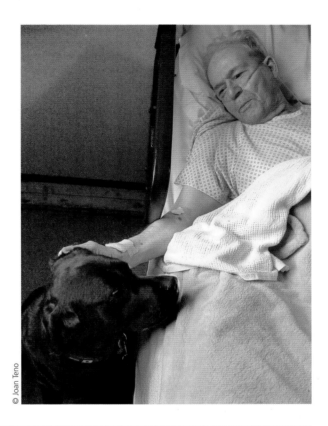

© Joan Teno

---

**Box 12.2. Controlling symptoms of terminal heart failure among very old people**

The Galliera Hospital in Genoa, Italy has introduced a palliative approach to caring for people with terminal heart failure in their unit for acute care for older people. The median age of the people residing in the unit is close to 90 years, and they generally have severe comorbidity and communication problems. Most have distressing symptoms in the terminal phase: breathlessness, agitation, death rattle, pain, nausea and vomiting. Most symptomatic patients have access to treatment on low-dose morphine (less than 20 mg per day on average) in combination with other medication (haloperidol, metoclopramide and scopolamine butylbromide). In the terminal phase, one third of the residents are severely distressed and agitated. They receive a slight increase in palliative drug dosages and/or low-dose midazolam for effective relief or sedation. This approach achieves acceptable symptom control in the dying process for older people with heart failure.

*Source*: personal communication, Vito Curiale, Galliera Hospital, Genoa, Italy.

## Box 12.3. Fighting polypharmacy

A team in Israel has developed novel procedures for improving drug therapy for frail older people. For each person, every medication is re-evaluated to decide whether to continue with the same dose, reduce it or discontinue it completely. Decisions are evidence-based wherever possible and otherwise based on clinical judgement. Using this procedure resulted in the discontinuation of an average of 2.8 drugs per person with no significant adverse effects. Mortality and referral rates to acute care facilities declined, and the cost of drugs dropped substantially.

The same practice and algorithm for drug discontinuation was found to be safe and effective among older people living in the community (average follow-up 19 months); 47% of all drugs were stopped (3.7 ± 2.5 drugs per participant), and successful discontinuation was eventually achieved among 81%. Drug discontinuation was not associated with significant adverse effects. Eighty per cent of the people discontinuing drugs and their families reported improvements in health, functioning, mental well-being and cognitive performance.

*Sources*: Garfinkel et al. *(7)* and Garfinkel *(8)*.

## References

1. Walsh D et al. *Palliative medicine*. New York, Saunders Elsevier, 2008.
2. Hanks G et al., eds. *Oxford textbook of palliative medicine*. 4th ed. Oxford, Oxford University Press, 2009.
3. Bruera E et al., eds. *Textbook of palliative medicine*. London, Hodder Arnold, 2006.
4. Solano JP, Gomes B, Higginson IJ. A comparison of symptom prevalence in far advanced cancer, AIDS, heart disease, chronic obstructive pulmonary disease and renal disease. *Journal of Pain and Symptom Management*, 2006, 31:58–69.
5. Seale C, Cartwright A. *The year before death*. London, Avebury Press, 1994.
6. American Geriatrics Society Panel on Persistent Pain in Older Persons. The management of persistent pain in older persons. *Journal of the American Geriatrics Society*, 2002, 50(Suppl.):S205–S224 (http://www.americangeriatrics.org/products/positionpapers/JGS5071.pdf, accessed 1 December 2010).
7. Garfinkel D, Zur-Gil S, Ben-Israel J. The war against polypharmacy: a new cost-effective geriatric-palliative approach for improving drug therapy in disabled elderly people. *Israel Medical Association Journal*, 2007, 9:430–434.
8. Garfinkel D. Symposium title: the war against polypharmacy rethinking and re-evaluation needed for each and every drug in the elderly (results of the good-palliative-geriatric-practice in the first 70 case reports). 19th World Congress of the International Association of Geriatrics & Gerontology (IAGG World) Congress of Gerontology & Geriatrics, Paris, 5–9 July 2009. Abstract book. *Journal of Nutrition, Health & Aging*, 2009, 13(Suppl. 1): SB7 116–4.
9. Lynch T et al. Barriers to the development of palliative care in the countries of central and eastern Europe and the Commonwealth of Independent States. *Journal of Pain and Symptom Management*, 2009, 37:305–315.
10. Kovach CR et al. Assessment and treatment of discomfort for people with late-stage dementia. *Journal of Pain and Symptom Management*, 1999, 18:412–419.

# 13

# Advance care planning

Advance care planning involves discussion about preferences for future care between an individual and a care provider in anticipation of future deterioration. These discussions may lead to several outcomes *(1)*, although slightly different terms may be used and the legal status of the statements varies.

- An advance statement: a statement of wishes and preferences setting out the person's general values and views about care. It is not legally binding.
- An advance decision to refuse treatment: involves refusal of a specific medical treatment in a predefined potential future situation. It is legally binding in some countries only if an individual loses capacity.
- Lasting power of attorney: involves appointing a person (an "attorney") to take decisions on behalf of an individual if they lose capacity to do so.

Older people may benefit from making advance statements, including reducing the burden of decision-making on their families, but they also have concerns about associations with euthanasia; the possibility that preferences for care may change; reluctance to think about death; and the time needed for older people to trust professionals enough to talk about such sensitive issues *(2)*. There are also concerns that such statements are nearly always about treatment withdrawal rather than specifying active choices, with the fear that this feeds into prejudice against age and disability *(3)*. Some doctors are unsure of the legal status of advance directives, which can result in them being misapplied or ignored *(4)*. Advance care planning has been used more extensively in North America and Canada than it has in Europe. However, a study of the effect of advance directives in Switzerland suggests that they might be useful in achieving improved communication, higher satisfaction with decision-making at the end of life and less anxiety and depression *(5)*. In general, older people may choose to undertake advance planning near to the time of disability and illness *(6)*.

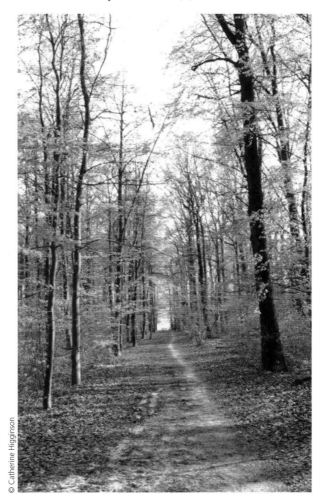
© Catherine Higginson

The application of advance care planning in countries in the European Region needs to be evaluated and must consider the different cultures and values, the terms used and the differences between health care systems when interpreting the evidence. For example, legislation in the United States of America requires that all individuals admitted to a care home be offered advance care planning. In addition to facilitating individual choice (Box 13.1), advance care planning may reduce the cost of health care at the end of life (Box 13.2).

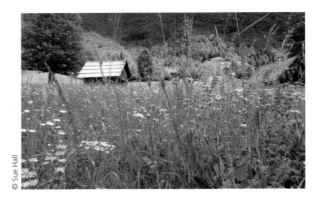

© Sue Hall

### Box 13.1. Preferred Priorities for Care in the United Kingdom

The Preferred Priorities for Care (7) is a document held by the person who is to receive care. It was developed in the United Kingdom and designed to facilitate choice in relation to end-of-life issues. People become empowered by sharing important information with all professionals involved in their care. The explicit recording of the wishes of people receiving care and their caregivers can form the basis of care planning in multidisciplinary teams and other services, minimizing inappropriate admissions and interventions. In care homes for older people, this is an opportunity for residents and staff to work together to develop advance care plans. Residents can initiate the plan at any time, and this will help staff members to follow their wishes and act as an advocate if the resident loses capacity towards the end of his or her life. Early evaluations suggest that such plans significantly influence people receiving care in their preferred place of care at the end of life, without significant changes in the services needed.

*Sources: The Preferred Priorities for Care (PPC) document: guidelines for health and/or social care staff (8) and Preferred Priorities for Care (9).*

### Box 13.2. Advance directives in nursing homes

Staff in local hospitals and nursing homes, residents and their families in Ontario, Canada were educated in advance planning. Three nurses from care homes attended a two-day workshop and then disseminated knowledge to other staff in the home. This resulted in fewer residents being sent to hospital and a reduction in the cost of hospital care from Can$ 1772 per resident in homes that used this approach versus Can$ 3869 homes not using it. Total health care and implementation costs were also lower: Can$ 3490 per resident versus Can$ 5239. This includes the cost for hospitalization, drugs and costs related to implementing the advance care planning.

*Source: Molloy et al. (10).*

## References

1. *Advance care planning: national guidelines*. London, Royal College of Physicians, 2009.
2. Seymour J et al. Planning for the end of life: the views of older people about advance care statements. *Social Science and Medicine*, 2004, 59:57–68.
3. O'Neill D. Present, rather than advance directives. *Lancet*, 2001, 358:1921–1922.
4. Toller CAS, House MS, Budge MM. Compliance with and understanding of advance directives among trainee doctors in the United Kingdom. *Journal of Palliative Care*, 2006, 22:141–146.
5. Pautex S, Herrmann FR, Zulian GB. Role of advance directives in palliative care units: a prospective study. *Palliative Medicine*, 2008, 22:835–841.
6. Garavan R et al. When and how older people discuss preferences for long-term care options. *Journal of the American Geriatrics Society*, 2009, 57:750–751.
7. Preferred Priorities for Care [web site]. Leicester, National End of Life Care Programme, National Health Service, 2010 (http://www.endoflifecareforadults.nhs.uk/eolc/ppc.htm, accessed 1 December 2010).
8. *The Preferred Priorities for Care (PPC) document: guidelines for health and/or social care staff*. Leicester, National End of Life Care Programme, National Health Service, 2007 (http://www.endoflifecareforadults.nhs.uk/eolc/files/F2111-PPC_Staff_Guidance_Dec2007.pdf, accessed 1 December 2010).
9. *Preferred Priorities for Care*. Leicester, National End of Life Care Programme, National Health Service, 2007 (http://www.endoflifecareforadults.nhs.uk/eolc/files/F2110-Preferred_Priorities_for_Care_V2_Dec2007.pdf, accessed 1 December 2010).
10. Molloy DW et al. Systematic implementation of an advance directive programme in nursing homes: a randomized control trial. *Journal of the American Medical Association*, 2000, 283:1437–1444.

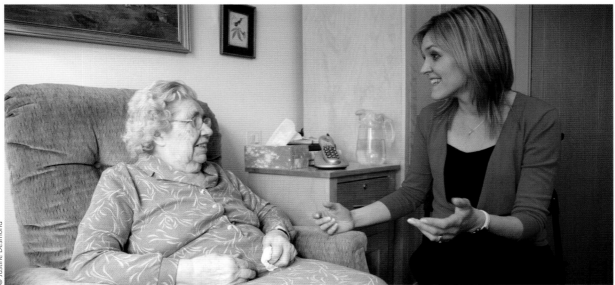

© Justine Desmond

# 14

# Integrated care pathways

Care pathways are structured multidisciplinary care plans that detail essential steps in the care of people with a specific clinical problem and describe their expected clinical course *(1)*.

They can provide a link between the establishment of clinical guidelines and their use and can help in communicating with the people who need care by giving them access to a clearly written summary of their expected care plan and progress over time. Care pathways can help promote teamwork and patient-centred care.

Such care pathways for palliative and end-of-life care have been developed in several countries, including for inpatients *(2)* and oncology units *(3)* in the United States of America and in other settings *(4)*.

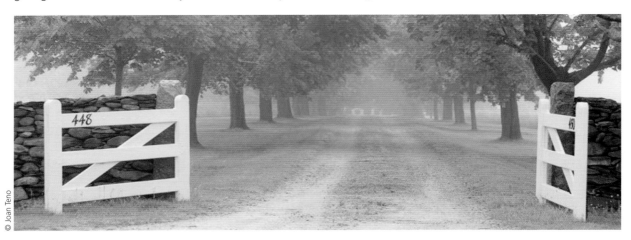

© Joan Teno

448

---

### Box 14.1. Liverpool Care Pathway for the Dying Patient

The Liverpool Care Pathway (LCP) has been developed in the United Kingdom to transfer the hospice model of care for people who are dying into other care settings *(5)*. The pathway has been modified for people with other conditions, such as kidney disease, heart failure and dementia *(6)* and has been successfully disseminated in 18 countries outside the United Kingdom. The LCP has been adapted to Australia's health care setting *(7)* and has been successfully implemented in the Hong Kong Special Administrative Region of China *(8)*. The LCP has been translated into Dutch and tested in three settings in the Netherlands: hospital, nursing homes and home care *(9)*. Everyone in the dying phase was put on the pathway. During the period when the pathway was being used, documentation of care was more comprehensive and there was a reduction in the symptoms as reported by staff or bereaved relatives. The LCP is now being tested for effectiveness in a multicentre randomized controlled trial in six regions of Italy.

*Source:* personal communication, Massimo Costantini, Regional Palliative Care Network, National Institute for Cancer Research, Genoa, Italy.

## References

1. Campbell H et al. Integrated care pathways. *British Medical Journal,* 1998, 316:133–137.

2. Bailey FA et al. Improving processes of hospital care during the last hours of life. *Archives of Internal Medicine,* 2005, 165:1722–1727.

3. Luhrs CA et al. Pilot of a pathway to improve the care of imminently dying oncology inpatients in a Veterans Affairs medical center. *Journal of Pain and Symptom Management,* 2005, 29:544–551.

4. Ellershaw J, Wilkinson S, eds. *Care of the dying: a pathway to excellence.* Oxford, Oxford University Press, 2003.

5. Liverpool Care Pathway for the Dying Patient (LCP) [web site]. Liverpool, Marie Curie Palliative Care Institute, 2010 (http://www.mcpcil.org.uk/liverpool-care-pathway/index.htm, accessed 1 December 2010).

6. McClelland B et al. *End-of-life care: an evaluation of the implementation of the Gold Standards Framework and the Liverpool Care Pathway for people with dementia in five care settings across Greater Manchester Evaluation Report. Executive summary.* London, Department of Health, 2008 (http://www.dhcarenetworks.org.uk/_library/Resources/Dementia/End_of_Life_Care_-_Evaluation_of_the_Implementation.pdf, accessed 1 December 2010).

7. Jackson K, Mooney C, Campbell D. The development and implementation of the pathway for improving the care of the dying in general medical wards. *Internal Medicine Journal,* 2009, 39:695–699.

8. Lo SH et al. The implementation of an end-of-life integrated care pathway in a Chinese population. *International Journal of Palliative Nursing,* 2009, 15:384–388.

9. Veerbeek L et al. The effect of the Liverpool Care Pathway for the dying: a multicentre study. *Palliative Medicine,* 2008, 22:145–151.

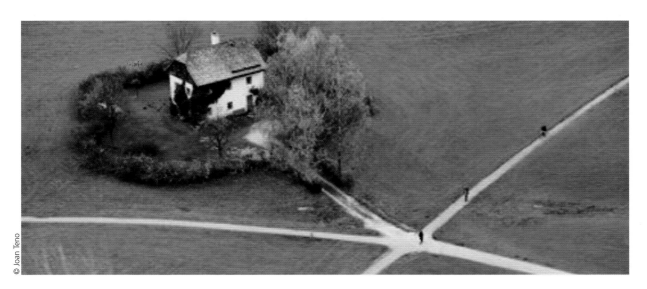

© Joan Teno

# 15

## Improving palliative care in resource-constrained settings

> "Palliative care is an urgent humanitarian need worldwide."
>
> *Source: Palliative care (1).*

There is unanimous agreement that good palliative care should reach everyone who needs it. Although providing examples of palliative care for older people in resource-constrained settings such as Africa is beyond the scope of this publication, including some reference to these settings is important for two main reasons.

First, these countries greatly need better palliative care. Second, the European Region can learn from some of the developments in resource-constrained settings, where much is achieved in the community on low budgets such as mobile hospices in Uganda (shown in photograph). Bus rounds could be a time-saving and cost-effective way of providing education in palliative care (Box 15.1).

Palliative care is an emerging discipline in Africa. Although there are centres of excellence providing holistic palliative care and education, these tend to be few and cannot currently provide enough palliative care to appropriately respond to the HIV epidemic, to progressive malignant disease and to the yet-unknown burden of non-malignant, non-HIV-related deaths. Research and auditing are essential to capture the lessons learned, to guide the wise allocation of scarce resources, to develop feasible and acceptable local models of palliative care and to ensure that people needing care and families in resource-constrained settings receive effective care. The example shown in Box 15.2 demonstrates the importance and feasibility of locally owned measurement and improvement of quality for people with progressive and advanced disease and their families in resource-constrained settings.

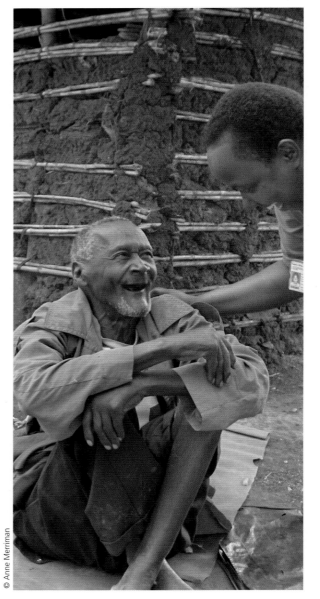

© Anne Merriman

## Box 15.1. Bus rounds as an educational tool in Argentina

Bus rounds by a group of specialist physicians and nurses were organized as part of a congress in Argentina to promote patient-based education of physicians and nurses. Specialist physicians and nurses visited people at home and in acute hospitals. To save time, the cases were presented and journal articles read during the bus journey. On average, five cases were presented during each round. The people receiving care and the specialist physicians and nurses were highly satisfied with bus rounds. They provided an opportunity for intensive exposure to patient-based learning both in hospitals and at home. The limited time spent in each home or hospice causes minimal disruption to the person and the family.

*Source*: Bruera et al. *(2)*.

## Box 15.2. Clinical auditing in Africa

A protocol for clinical auditing in palliative care in sub-Saharan Africa has been developed in the United Kingdom. Researchers are working in partnership with African palliative care providers and advocates to facilitate the measurement and improvement of care *(3)*. The ENCOMPASS protocol (Ensuring Core Outcomes and Measuring Palliation in Sub-Saharan Africa) is a two-year project based on collaboration between five of the leading palliative care providers in South Africa and Uganda, King's College London and Cicely Saunders International. The collaboration ensures that each setting is able to coordinate its own quality improvement strategy and set it its own targets relevant to its own facility. Each centre works with its multiprofessional clinical teams to measure patient and family outcomes using the African version of the Palliative Care Outcome Scale *(4,5)*, to reflect on its own data, to set quality improvement targets, to devise clinical training and responses to meet these targets, to implement its strategies and to measure change with the aim to determine whether targets had been met.

*Source*: personal communication, Richard Harding, King's College London, United Kingdom.

## References

1. *Palliative care*. Geneva, World Health Organization, 2007 (Cancer control: knowledge into action: WHO guide for effective programmes, Module 5; http://www.who.int/cancer/media/FINAL-Palliative%20Care%20Module.pdf, accessed 1 December 2010).
2. Bruera E et al. Bus rounds for medical congresses on palliative care. *Supportive Care in Cancer*, 1998, 6:529–532.
3. *Measuring patient and family outcomes in palliative care in Africa*. Kampala, African Palliative Care Association, 2010 (http://www.apca.co.ug/opinions/Measuring20patient%20and%20family%20outcomes.htm, accessed 1 December 2010).
4. *Newsletter 3: spring*. London, Cicely Saunders International, 2008.
5. Powell RA et al. Development of the APCA African Palliative Outcome Scale. *Journal of Pain and Symptom Management*, 2007, 33:229–232.

# 16

## The need for research on palliative care for older people

> "Palliative medicine is a rapidly evolving field, which is quickly moving to redress its historical paucity of high-quality research evidence."
>
> *Source*: Currow et al. *(1)*.

This publication includes examples of innovative approaches to improve palliative care for older people. Since many of these have not been rigorously evaluated, they can best be described as emerging or promising rather than best practices. Research in palliative care has been described as small and descriptive, lacking the quality to contribute to evidence-based medicine *(2)*. This is partly due to the lack of dedicated research funding and academic positions in palliative care in most countries in the European Region. There are also challenges to conducting research on palliative care, such as ethical concerns about placing an extra burden on the people needing care and their families and high attrition rates in longitudinal studies due to deterioration in people's condition.

High-quality research is urgently needed on palliative care in general and especially on palliative care for older people. Given the limited health budgets in most countries, such research needs to include information on the cost–effectiveness of treatment and services.

In recent years, several research initiatives have emerged in Europe and North America.

- In Canada, Can$ 16.5 million was allocated to a palliative care initiative, with a substantial amount allocated to research grants. A specific palliative care research panel has been established.
- The United States of America has a National Palliative Care Research Center.
- In the United Kingdom, the Department of Health has established a national framework for cancer research. The National Cancer Research Network has a group on clinical studies of palliative care to facilitate the development of new clinical trials and funds, and the National Cancer Research Institute has set up two supportive and palliative care research collaboratives to foster more collaboration and interdisciplinary work: Cancer Experiences Collaborative *(3)* and COMPASS Collaborative *(4)*.
- In Europe, a European Association for Palliative Care Research Network was established in 1996. The European Association for Palliative Care and the International Association for Hospice and Palliative Care joined forces with other regional and academic organisations to initiate a global

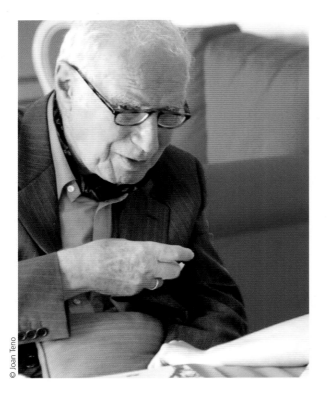

© Joan Teno

palliative care research initiative with a special focus on low- and medium-income countries. Many organizations have signed the Declaration of Venice: Palliative Care Research in Developing Countries *(5)* to support this initiative, and the EU has funded major programmes to foster research collaboration across Europe (Boxes 16.1–16.4).

- The world's first purpose-built institute of palliative care has been opened at King's College London. The Cicely Saunders Institute was designed with patient and family involvement and seeks to integrate research, education, clinical care and the provision of information and support *(6)*.

These and future research initiatives are essential if palliative care is to continue to evolve.

Palliative care streams funded internationally by the EU and nationally in individual countries are needed. Given the ageing of the population in the European Region, this should include a focus on meeting the palliative care needs of older people. Effective collaboration between palliative care and geriatrics along with translational research is needed to achieve this. Future researchers also need to consider the ability to generalize their findings and provide the necessary information to assist clinicians, health planners and funders in applying palliative care research in real-world settings *(2)*.

### Box 16.1. European Palliative Research Collaborative

The European Palliative Research Collaborative *(7)*, consisting of eight participating centres from six European countries, was funded for three years. The aim was to develop novel genetic methods for predicting responses to opioids, individual variation of cachexia and methods for assessing and classifying pain and cachexia. The objectives were: to identify people at particular risk for developing cachexia; to improve the classification and assessment of pain, depression and cachexia; develop an Internet-based system for implementing European evidence-based guidelines; and to develop a long-lasting European collaborative in palliative care cancer research.

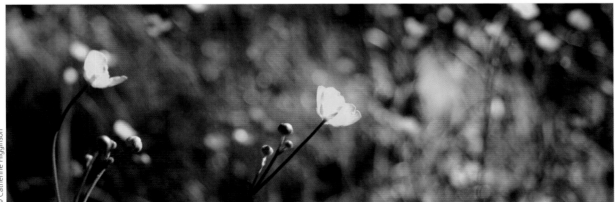

© Catherine Higginson

3. Invest in research, development and education as part of the overall strategy on palliative care for older people.
4. Plan palliative care for older people at the level of local government and develop strategies that promote effective leadership and community action in planning and implementing care, consistent with the culture of the community organization and its norms, standards and organizational structure: a single provider, separation between health and social care or separation of responsibilities at different government levels depending on the type of health care system.

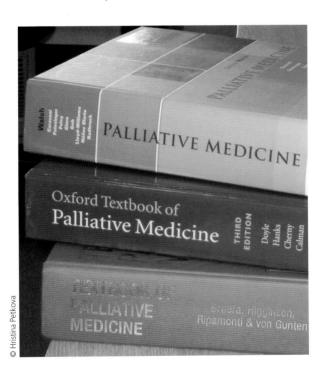

© Hristina Petkova

## Health professionals need to do the following.

1. Ensure they are adequately trained and up to date in both geriatrics and the palliative care of older people, including assessing and treating pain and other symptoms, communication skills and coordination of care.
2. Measure the outcomes of their routine care regularly, including for older people.
3. Ensure that older people with palliative care needs are regarded as individuals, that their right to make decisions about their health and social care is respected and that they receive the unbiased information they need without experiencing discrimination because of their age.
4. Ensure that their organizations work in coordination and collaboration with other statutory, private or voluntary organizations that may provide help or services for older people needing palliative care.
5. Participate in research, education and auditing that seek to improve palliative care.

## Those funding research should do the following.

1. Invest in programmes that develop and robustly determine the effectiveness and cost-effectiveness of ways to improve palliative care for older people, including people with diseases other than cancer. These programmes should be sustained over a period of time so that new models of care and interventions can be developed and evaluated.
2. Promote collaboration in comparing best practices in palliative care in various countries.

3. Invest in creative research into the barriers to accessing palliative care, the origin and management of pain in diseases other than cancer and other symptoms older people have, their subjective experience of care, the mental and social needs of different cultural groups, the testing of advance care planning and meeting the needs of frail older people.

4. Promote collaboration in research between palliative care and geriatric medicine, geriatric nursing and mental health services for older people and the inclusion of older people in all kinds of innovative research on physical interventions, including drug treatment.

5. Disseminate the findings of research on palliative care for older people and constantly review the uptake.

6. Monitor the proportion of funds in any disease or subject area that is directed towards palliative care research, especially that involving older people, and invest in redressing imbalances.

7. Encourage innovative research (ideas that are most likely to make a difference in practice) to help people with serious chronic illnesses to live well and die well.

8. Invest in methodological development in palliative care research among older people, especially among groups that are difficult to reach, including residents of nursing homes.

9. Ensure that experts with relevant expertise assess research on palliative care among older people.

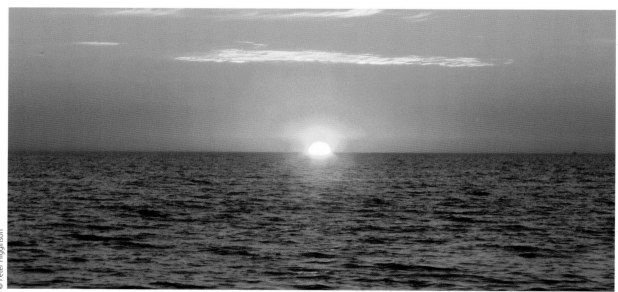

© Peter Higginson

# Annex 1. Wider consultation group

A draft of this publication was sent to the following experts, many of whom made extremely helpful comments.

**Australia**
Ian Maddocks
School of Medicine, Flinders University of South Australia, Adelaide
Deborah Parker
School of Nursing and Midwifery, University of Queensland

**Austria**
Herbert Watzke
Unit of Palliative Care, Medical University of Vienna,
and Austrian Palliative Care Study Group
Franz Zdrahal
Austrian Society of Palliative Care, Caritas of Vienna

**Belgium**
Anne-Marie De Lust
Federation Palliative Care Flanders, Wemmel
Tine de Vlieger
Palliatieve Hulpverlening Antwerpen, Wilrijk
Anne-Françoise Nollet
Federation of Palliative Care for Wallonia, Namur
Bart Van den Eynden
Centre for Palliative Care Sint-Camillus, University of Antwerp

**Bosnia and Herzegovina**
Adnan Delibegovic
Department of Palliative Care, Tuzla
and Sarajevo Association for Palliative Care

**Bulgaria**
Nikolay Radev Yordanov
Department of Palliative Care, Interregional Cancer Hospital,
Vratsa and Bulgarian Association for Palliative Care

**Canada**
Kevin Brazil
McMaster University, St. Joseph's Health System Research Network, Ontario
Albert J. Kirshen
Temmy Latner Centre for Palliative Care, Toronto

**China, Hong Kong Special Administrative Region**
Sian Griffiths
School of Public Health and Primary Care,
Chinese University of Hong Kong
Mok Chun Keung
Consultant Geriatrician, Tuen Mun Hospital

**Croatia**
Maja Boban
Croatian Society for Hospice/Palliative Care
Marijana Bras
President, Croatian Medical Association;
Croatian Society for Hospice/Palliative Care
Juliana Franinovic-Markovic
Palliative Care Unit, Rijeka

Anica Jusic
Croatian Society for Hospice and Palliative Care, Zagreb
Ivanka Kotnik
Croatian Association of Hospice Friends
Gordana Spoljar
President, Croatian Association of Hospice Friends
Ana Stambuk
Faculty of Law, Zagreb

**Cyprus**
Anna Achilleoudi
President, Cyprus Association of Cancer Patients
and Cyprus Cancer Prevention and Palliative Care
Jane Kakas
Cyprus Association of Cancer Patients and Friends, Limassol
Sophia Pantekhi
Cyprus Anti-Cancer Society, Arodaphnousa
Evdokimos Xenophontos
President, Cyprus Anti-Cancer Society

**Denmark**
Bodil Abild Jespersen
Aarhus University Hospital/Aarhus Palliative Team
Per Sjøgren
Unit of Palliative Medicine, Pain Centre, Rigshospitalet
Copenhagen University Hospital

**Finland**
Tiina Saarto
Department of Oncology, Helsinki University Central Hospital,
and Finnish Association for Palliative Medicine
Mikaela von Bonsdorff
Department of Health Sciences, Finnish Centre for Interdisciplinary
Gerontology, University of Jyväskylä, Viveca

**France**
Jacqueline Bories
Société Française d'Accompagnement et SP, Paris
Marilene Filbet
Hospices Civils de Lyon, Centre de Soins Palliatifs, Lyon
Godefroy Hirsch
President, Société Française d'Accompagnement de Soins Palliatifs SFAP
Claude Jasmin
International Council for Global Health Progress, Hôpital Paul Brousse, Villejuif
Aude Le Devinah
Ministry of Health, Paris
Paulette Le Lann
Fédération Jusqu'à la Mort Accompagner la Vie (JALMALV); IRFAC, Rouen
Wadih Rhondali
Hospices Civils de Lyon, Centre de Soins Palliatifs, Lyon
Christophe Trivalle
Hôpital Paul Brousse, Villejuif
Chantal Wood
Unité d'Evaluation et de Traitement de la Hôpital Robert Debré

**Germany**
Eberhard Klaschik
Centre for Palliative Medicine, University of Bonn,
Deutsche Gesellschaft für Palliativmedizin
Christof Müller-Busch
President, Deutsche Gesellschaft für Palliativmedizin
Friedemann Nauck
Department of Palliative Care, Medical University of Göttingen
Thomas Schindler
Nord-Rhein-Westfalen, Geldern

**Greece**
Kyriaki Mystakidou
President, Hellenic Association for Pain Control & Palliative Care;
University of Athens
Athina Vadalouca
President, Hellenic Society of Palliative & Symptomatic Care of Cancer
and Non-Cancer Patients; Areteion Hospital, Athens

**Hungary**
Katalin Hegedus
Hungarian Hospice Palliative Association; Semmelweis University,
Institute of Behavioural Sciences, Budapest

**Ireland**
Phil Larkin
University College Dublin/Our Lady's Hospice
Julie Ling
Department of Health and Children, Dublin
Avril O'Sullivan
Irish Cancer Society, Dublin
Karen Ryan
St Francis Hospice, Mater Misericordiae University Hospital
and Connolly Hospital, Dublin

**Israel**
Michaela Bercovitch
Sheba Medical Center Oncological Hospice;
President, Israel Palliative Medical Society
Doron Garfinkel
Geriatric Palliative Department, Shoham Geriatric Medical Center, Pardes Hana
Yoram Singer
President, Israel Association of Palliative Care

**Italy**
Roberto Bernabei
Centro Medicina Invecchiamento, Università Cattolica del Sacro Cuore, Rome
Augusto Caraceni
Virgilio Floriani Hospice, Palliative Care Unit, National Cancer Institute, Milan
Franco De Conno
Istituto Nazionale per lo Studio e la Cura dei Tumori, Milan
Francesca Crippa Floriani
President, Federazione Cure Palliative Onlus
Claude Fusco-Karman
Lega Italiana per la Lotta contro i Tumori, Milan
Daisy Maitilasso
Società Italiana di Cure Palliative, Milan

Carla Ripamonti,
Istituto Nazionale per lo Studio e la Cura dei Tumori, Milan
Franco Toscani,
Istituto Maestroni Istituto di Ricerca in Medicina Palliativa Onlus, Cremona
Giovanni Zaninetta,
President, Società Italiana di Cure Palliative

**Latvia**
Vilnis Sosars
President, Palliative Care Association of Latvia

**Lithuania**
Arvydas Seskevicius
Lithuanian Palliative Medicine Association

**Netherlands**
Arianne Brinkman-Stoppelenburg
Netherlands Palliative Care Network for Terminally Ill Patients
Luc Deliens
End-of-Life Care Research Group, Vrije Universiteit Brussel;
Department of Public and Occupational Health, EMGO Institute for Health
and Care Research, VU University Medical Centre, Amsterdam
André Rhebergen
Agora Ondersteuningspunt Palliatieve, Agora
Miel Ribbe
VU University Medical Centre, Amsterdam
Frans Van Soest
President, Netherlands Palliative Care Network for Terminally Ill Patients

**Norway**
Eva Albert
Norwegian Association for Palliative Medicine
Dagny Faksvag Haugen
Haukeland University Hospital, Bergen
Britta Hjertaas
Norwegian Palliative Association
Bodil Husby
Norwegian Palliative Association
Jon Håvard Loge
Norwegian Association for Palliative Medicine
Lotte Rogg
Norwegian Association for Palliative Medicine

**Portugal**
Edna Goncalves
Serviço de Cuidados Paliativos do Hospital Central Universitario de São João,
Porto, and Portuguese Association of Palliative Care
Isabel Galriça Neto
President, Portuguese Association of Palliative Care
Silvia Pereira
Portuguese Association of Palliative Care

**Romania**
Constantin Bogdan
Romanian Society of Palliatology & Thanatology
Daniela Mosoiu
Asociatia Nationala de Ingrijiri Paliative

**Romania (continued)**
Anca Pantea
Asociatia Nationala de Ingrijiri Paliative
Gabriela Rahnea-Nita
St Luca Hospital, Bucharest

**Serbia**
Natasa Milicevic
Centre for Palliative Care and Palliative Medicine, "Belhospice", Belgrade

**Slovenia**
Urska Lunder
Palliative Care Development Institute, Ljubljana

**Spain**
Carlos Centeno
Equipo de Medicina Paliativa Clínica Universitaria,
Universidad de Navarra, Pamplona
Javier Rocafort Gil
Spanish Society of Palliative Care
Xavier Gómez-Batiste
Director, WHO Collaborating Centre for Public Health Palliative Care
Programmes; and the "QUALY" End of Life Observatory;
Hospital Duran i Reynals, Institut Català d'Oncologia, Barcelona
Maria Nabal
Hospital Universitario Arnau de Vilanova, Lerida
Jordi Roca
Hospital de la Santa Creu, Barcelona
Jose Espinosa Rojas
Centre Collaborador OMS per Programes Públics de Cures Palliatives,
Observatori Fi de Vida de Catalunya, Institut Català d'Oncologia,
Barcelona
Carme Sala Rovira
Soc. Catalano-Balear de Cures Palliatives

**Sweden**
Maria Jakobsson
Swedish Association for Palliative Medicine
Gunilla Lundquist
Swedish Association for Palliative Medicine
Sylvia Sauter
Swedish Council for Palliative Care
Peter Strang
Karolinska Institute, Stockholm
Carol Tishelman
Karolinska Institute, Stockholm
Eva Thoren Todoulos
Swedish Association for Palliative Medicine

**Switzerland**
Laura Di Pollina
Clinical Geriatrics, Geneva University Hospitals
Steffen Eychmüller
Cantonal Hospital St. Gallen, St. Gallen;
Société Suisse de Médecine et de Soins Palliatifs
Roland Kunz
Société Suisse de Médecine et de Soins Palliatifs

Sophie Pautex
Service of Palliative Medicine, Department of Rehabilitation and Geriatrics,
Geneva University Hospitals, Geneva
Mathias Pfisterer
European Union Geriatric Medicine Society; Department of Cardiology,
University Hospital, Basel

**Uganda**
Godfrey Agupio
Hospice Africa, Uganda
Anne Merriman
Hospice Africa, Uganda

**Ukraine**
Vladyslav Mykhalskyy
Ukraine Association of Palliative Care and Minimally Invasive Therapy

**United Kingdom**
Julia Addington-Hall
Research Group Cancer, Palliative & End of Life Care,
School of Health Sciences, University of Southampton
Simon Biggs
Institute of Gerontology, King's College London
Harry Cayton
Macmillan Cancer Support
Simon Chapman
National Council for Palliative Care, London
David Clark
Lancaster University; International Observatory on End of Life Care
Jessica Corner
Macmillan Cancer Support
Deirdre Cunningham
South East London Strategic Health Authority
Ciarán Devane
Macmillan Cancer Support
Ilora Finlay
University Medical School of Wales, Cardiff
Pam Firth
Isabel Hospice, Hertfordshire
Katherine Froggatt
Division of Health Research, School of Health and Medicine, Lancaster University
Geoffrey Hanks
Bristol Haematology and Oncology Centre, Department of Palliative Medicine
Lynne Hargreaves
International Observatory on End of Life Care
Claire Henry
National End of Life Care Strategy (England)
Jo Hockley
Palliative Care and Care Homes Network
Andrew Hoy
Princess Alice Hospice, Surrey
Tom Hughes-Hallett
Marie Curie Cancer Care, London
Rowena Jackson
International Observatory on End of Life Care
Bridget Johnston
Palliative Care Research Society

**United Kingdom (continued)**
Marilyn Kendall
Palliative Care Research Society Ross Lawrenson, University of Surrey,
Guildford; and University of Auckland
Jane Maher
Macmillan Cancer Support
Martin McKee
London School of Hygiene and Tropical Medicine
Thomas William Noble
Association for Palliative Medicine of Great Britain and Ireland
Sheila Payne
Lancaster University; Division of Health Research,
International Observatory on End of Life Care
Michael Pearson
Royal College of Physicians, London
David Prail
Help the Hospices, London
Mike Richards
Department of Health, London
Stephen Richards
Macmillan Cancer Support
Eve Richardson
National Council for Palliative Care, London
Jane Seymour
University of Nottingham
Gail Sharp
Marie Curie Cancer Care, London
Sue Smith
Association of Palliative Care Social Workers
Les Storey
Preferred Priorities for Care
Peter Tebbit
National Council for Palliative Care, London
Keri Thomas
Gold Standards Framework
John Wiles
Association for Palliative Medicine of Great Britain and Ireland
Alison Woodbridge-Nash
Association of Palliative Care Social Workers

**United States of America**
Mary Callaway
Open Society Institute, New York, NY
David Caseratt
University of Pennsylvania, Philadelphia, PA

Christine Cassel
American Board of Internal Medicine, Philadelphia, PA
Frank Ferris
San Diego Hospice and the Institute for Palliative Medicine, San Diego, CA
Kathleen M. Foley
Memorial Sloan-Kettering Cancer Center, New York, NY
Karl Lorenz
Veterans Integrated Palliative Program, Veterans Affairs
Greater Los Angeles Healthcare System, VA Palliative Care
Quality Improvement Resource Center, Los Angeles, CA
Joanne Lynn
Washington Home Center for Palliative Care Studies
and RAND Health, Washington, DC
David Mechanic
Institute for Health, Health Care Policy and Aging Research,
Rutgers University, New Brunswick, New Jersey
Diane E. Meier
Mount Sinai School of Medicine, New York, NY
Richard Della Penna
Kaiser Permanente Aging Network, San Diego, CA
Greg Sachs
Indiana University School of Medicine, Indianapolis, IN;
National Palliative Care Research Center

**WHO**
Enis Baris
Former Director, Division of Country Health Systems,
WHO Regional Office for Europe
Martina Pellny
Former Programme Manager, Division of Country Health Systems,
WHO Regional Office for Europe

**Administrators in these organizations and others who helped in
forwarding the document**
Heidi Blumhuber
European Association for Palliative Care
Amelia Giordano
European Association for Palliative Care
Avril Jackson
Help the Hospices, London
Sheila Joseph
National Programme Manager, National End of Life
Care Programme (England), Leicester
Jackie Main
National End of Life Care Programme (England), Leicester